The New
Speaking of Sex

Praise for Meg Hickling

Speaking of Sex *is a wonderful book for parents on how to answer children's questions about sex.* – THE PROVINCE

British Columbia's leading advocate for providing reproductive health information from kindergarten upward. – THE NATIONAL POST

Meg Hickling has a mission: to provide elementary school children with information about their own bodies – information that could save their lives. – VANCOUVER SUN

One of the many strengths of Hickling's book is the way she decodes the messages implicit in the things children ask. She shows parents how they can honor the question, react non-judgmentally, calmly provide factual information, and leave the door open for their kids to ask, or tell, what they need. – TIMES COLONIST

This is an extremely useful, often moving, and important book. It ought to come, at birth, with every child. – THE GEORGIA STRAIGHT

We've come a long way, thanks to the efforts of Meg Hickling.
– THE DAILY COURIER

MEG HICKLING RN

THE NEW

Speaking
OF sex

REVISED AND
UPDATED

WHAT YOUR CHILDREN NEED TO KNOW
AND WHEN THEY NEED TO KNOW IT

Northstone

Editor: Michael Schwartzentruber
Cover and interior design: Margaret Kyle
Cover artwork: Kim La Fave, Roberts Creek, BC, k_lafave@dccnet.com
Proofreading: Dianne Greenslade

Northstone Publishing acknowledges the financial support of the Government of Canada,
through the Book Publishing Industry Development Program, for its publishing activities.

NORTHSTONE PUBLISHING is an imprint of
WOOD LAKE BOOKS INC., an employee-owned company, and is committed to caring
for the environment and all creation. Northstone recycles, reuses, and composts, and
encourages readers to do the same. Resources are printed on recycled paper and more
environmentally friendly groundwood papers (newsprint), whenever possible. The trees
used are replaced through donations to the Scoutrees for Canada program.
A percentage of all profit is donated to charitable organizations.

Library and Archives Canada Cataloguing in Publication
Hickling, Meg, 1941-
The new speaking of sex: what your children need to know and
when they need to know it/Meg Hickling. – Rev. and updated
First ed. published 1996 under title: Speaking of sex.
2nd ed. published 1999 under title: More speaking of sex.
Includes bibliographical references and index.
ISBN 1-896836-70-4
1. Sex instruction for children. 2. Sex instruction for teenagers.
3. Family life education. I. Hickling, Meg, 1941- . More speaking of sex. II. Title.
HQ57.H53 2005   649'.65   C2004-906375-8

Published by Northstone Publishing,
an imprint of Wood Lake Books Inc.
Kelowna, BC, Canada
woodlakebooks.com

Printing 9 8 7 6 5 4 3 2 1

Printed in Canada by
Transcontinental Printing

Dedication

This book is respectfully dedicated to *all my students:*
to the children and teens who
taught me so much about their worlds;
to the thousands of parents who have shared their stories; and
to all the professionals who have been in my seminars
and not only told me how much they learned, but
who supported and encouraged my work.
And to *Sally McRae*, who first suggested that
the stories would make a book!

Contents

Foreword 9

Preface 11

Preface to the First Edition................................. 14

PART ONE
WHAT YOUR CHILDREN NEED TO KNOW AND WHEN THEY NEED TO KNOW IT

1. Let's Talk.. 21
2. Preschoolers: Magical Thinkers (Ages Two – Four) 35
3. Primaries: The Bathroom Humor Types
   (First Grade – Third Grade)... 57
4. Intermediates: The "Gross-me-outers"
   (Fourth Grade – Seventh Grade)................................... 75
5. Adolescents: The People Who Don't Know That
   They Don't Know (Seventh Grade – Twelfth Grade) 105
6. The Sexually Mature Adult.. 123
7. Alternate Ways to Get Pregnant................................. 133

PART TWO
STRAIGHT ANSWERS TO THE QUESTIONS YOUR CHILDREN WILL ASK

8. Straight Answers to the Questions Your Children Will Ask 143

PART THREE
HELPING YOUR CHILDREN STAY HEALTHY

9. The Sexually Active Teen 169
10. Sexually Transmitted Diseases (STDs) 177
11. What Happens in the Doctor's Office 189

PART FOUR
COMMUNICATING YOUR VALUES

12. Family Values 199
13. Parents and Families Who Are Faithful 211

PART FIVE
FOR EDUCATORS AND OTHER PROFESSIONALS

14. Sexual-Health Education in a Multicultural Society 223

Conclusion: Celebrating Diversity 229
Resources/Bibliography 231
Index 245

Foreword

How fortunate we are to live in a time when we know so much more, scientifically speaking, than generations preceding us! In the second edition of *Speaking of Sex*, author, lecturer, mother, wife, and nurse Meg Hickling continued to share the "latest and greatest" information about sexual health. This more comprehensive edition explores new trends, addresses common myths, discusses the impact of the Internet and pornography, and has a new chapter on sexual-health education in a multicultural society.

She gently dispels misconceptions and unhealthy beliefs about sex by telling even more humorous stories from over 20 years of experience working with children, families, teachers, and other professionals.

What I like most about *Speaking of Sex* is Meg's "whole person" approach to sex. She touches on the physical, intellectual, emotional, and spiritual aspects of sexuality. Using the notion of sexual health education as a "stretchable thing," she helps us stretch our own knowledge so that we might help children stretch theirs as they grow.

Meg assists us in our endeavors to educate our children about abuse, unplanned pregnancy, and sexually transmitted diseases (STDs), including HIV/AIDS. She gives us age-appropriate information, guidelines on how to talk with children at various stages of their development, and examples of how to answer tough questions.

What a wonderful, healthy community, sexually speaking, we could have if the attitudes and information shared by Meg became the norm in our society.

With humor, wit, and grace, Meg shares the gift of herself and her life experiences with us. My family, my patients, and my students and I are immensely grateful.

Dr. Margaret K. Merrifield, M.D., C.C.F.P.
Adolescent and Women's Health Care,
Physicians Medical Center
author of *Come Sit By Me* and *Morning Light*

Preface

S ince *Speaking of Sex* was first published in 1996, I have met many people who have expressed their thanks for all they have learned from the book. Most of us can be "stuck" at the adolescent level from time to time, believing that we know everything, especially since we are now parents, even grand- and great-grandparents.

Parents who are doctors and nurses have said, "Yes, the hardest people to talk to are my own." But even if it is easier to talk to your sister's children than your own, you force yourself to talk at home and, more importantly, you support any sexual health education that is offered in schools, faith groups, and community groups. Children and teens often say to me, "Oh yeah, my mom or my dad said that too." Suddenly, parents are looking pretty smart after all.

In the autumn of 1998, the United Nations published the results of a study done around the world and said sexual health education tends to encourage students to wait have sex until they are older. The report also said that students who have had sexual health education have fewer partners, fewer unplanned pregnancies, and fewer sexually transmitted diseases than those who have not had this kind of education.

Why did you pick this job out of all the jobs in the world???????

This study, I believe, makes even more evident the important role families have to play. Schools are not always able to provide complete education; it must be reinforced at home. Encourage yourself to use a light tone whenever possible, use humor and every listening skill you possess to get your family talking about sex!

Children are often much more knowledgeable and at ease than we expect and they can be surprisingly helpful during our own struggles. Let me tell you about one mom's conversation with her nine-year-old who was reading the sex advice column in her mother's magazine.

"Mom, what is oral sex?"

Trying hard not to show shock and panic, her mom replied, "Let's think like scientists. What does the word oral mean?"

"Oral means to do with the mouth," replied the daughter, thoughtfully. Then her face brightened and she said very matter-of-factly, "Oh, they mean a blow job! Why didn't they say so," and turned the page to a cookie recipe she wanted to try.

Even young students demonstrate a greater exposure to sexuality these days. I walked into a third grade classroom recently and just as I was beginning to introduce myself and the "body science" topic to the class, one young boy raised his hand and said very loudly, "I want to know first, what is foreplay?"

His poor teacher put his head in his hands and murmured, "Oh, Tim."

do you enjoy teaching people (kid's) about sex, pubirty and "private parts?"

The other students glanced at the teacher, but then calmly back at me.

"Well," I began, "let's think like scientists. Does everyone know that adults like to hug and kiss before they have sex?"

"Yes!" they all chorused, with a few "It's gross!" thrown in, naturally.

"Well," I continued, "if adults hug and kiss and *then* have sex, it's called foreplay."

Quite properly, one student then asked, "And if it is just hugging and no sex, then it is not foreplay?" What a brilliant scientist!

I can't say it often enough: this is lifesaving information. Your child really wants to ask these questions and they want to hear the answers from you. Never miss a teachable moment. Celebrate them.

Preface to the First Edition

This book is meant to illustrate my experience. It is not meant to be prescriptive. I hope that it will inspire readers to find their own truth.

The science and health information in this book also comes from my experience as a sexual health educator for over 20 years. It is not meant to be a medical text. Please consult your doctor if you have questions.

The stories and anecdotes in this book are true and I have tried to relate them as they were told to me or as I experienced them myself. Most stories, however, are not unique. In some instances, therefore, I have combined elements from various, similar stories into a single story.

How long did it take you to learn this stuff,

Every child and teen question that is reproduced in this book is as it was anonymously given to me in a class or group. I truly appreciate my students' honesty and openness in asking their questions. None of the questions reproduced here have been asked of me only once, and many of them have been asked dozens of times. They were chosen for inclusion in the book because of how common the question is or because of the poignancy and serious worry they express. I hope that everyone who reads the book can understand and accept the reality of the questions.

My professional life divides itself quite neatly into thirds. I spend one third of my time talking to "children" aged three to 93, in preschools to university classes. Another third is spent in meetings and workshops with parents, teaching them the skills to educate their children at home. The final third is spent with professionals who work with children: doctors, nurses, teachers, social workers, clergy, lawyers, pharmacists, and youth care workers.

When I first began teaching in 1974, it was just to parents and professionals about how to talk with children about sexual health. Then parents began to say, "Okay, Meg, you have convinced me that I should be talking to my children, but could you come over to my house Saturday morning and get me started?"

That request started "The Family Sessions." Following a two-hour seminar for the parents on how to talk at home, the parents then return on another evening and bring their children. We divide the evening into two sessions; one for primaries and their parents, and one for intermediates and their parents.

The children sit on the floor in front of me and the parents sit behind (they are on chairs). The parents listen as I present sexual health information to their children. The presentation is primarily for the parents; I model one way of talking to children about "body science." Afterward, the whole family goes home with common knowledge.

Parents have told me it becomes a wonderful reminder; years after the presentation, both parents and child have said, "What did Meg say about that?" And I love it when I hear the children say at the end of a family session, "Now I feel safe in the world, 'cuz I know my mom and dad know what I know." The adults are amazed at how much they learned. So are the students who didn't really want to come. They love the jokes and humor I use and despite their oft-repeated protests of "I know it all," they join in the discussion, ask questions, and share their stories. Thousands of preteens (and some early teens) have been frog marched into a family session, but none that I know of have gone home mad. "It was kinda gross, but good," is a comment I often hear.

Many parents now want me in the classrooms talking to the whole school and they even do the fundraising to pay for it. Others are satisfied with the family sessions.

The professional workshops contain information on the stages of sexual development in children, but also on what we call, "the latest and greatest information about sexual health." This includes information on STDs (sexually transmitted diseases), contraceptives, and the newest trends in issues and questions that children and teens are expressing. Many professionals have a dozen areas to keep up-to-date on, so they find these presentations extremely helpful.

I have been deeply honored to receive several awards and many of these professionals have supported my work and helped to nominate me for them. I would especially like to thank Shelly Rivkin, Roseann Farndon Lyster, Dan Marriott, Lynn Smith, Chris Simmons-Physick, Frances Kolotyluck, Greg Nicholson, George Alliston, Miriam Mauer, Arlene Burdon, Ian Hayson, Jeanne Fike, Maria LeRose, Adair Hobson, Donna Moyer, Rita Clarkson, Catherine Smailes, Barb Stoddard, Judy Gunderson, Sharon Connaughty, Sheila MacFarlane, and Pat Lauridsen-Hoegh.

There are, of course, many other people I would like to acknowledge. My dad, Bob Burtch, a Victorian gentleman of the first order, gave me permission to consider such a project by saying, "You should write those stories in a book."

I think that this program is important because it can save peoples lives.

My early teaching experiences were tremendously supported by other nurses and educators: Barb Hestrin, Mary Schmok, Maggie Pickering, Sandra Good, Laurie Kalbach, Linda Jones, Philippa Chicquen, June Pepin, Barbara Emmerson, Elizabeth Thomas, Kathleen Gauley, Pat Ward, Karen Lam, Brad Watson, Marcie Summers, and especially my long-time colleague and friend, Alice Bell. Some of my best lines have come from Alice and my wonderful sister, Bobbie Tough.

The importance of seeing sexuality and spirituality as one was taught to me by Glen and Patricia Baker, George Hermanson, Anne and George Searcy, as well as by John Cobb and David Schnarch.

I want to be the first to acknowledge that I am not everyone's "cup of tea." Some people heartily dislike me, my message, and my style of teaching. But I want to thank those who, in spite of their personal reservations, have had the courtesy to talk to me. Sometimes my greatest learnings have come from my harshest critics.

Writing a book has often been compared to giving birth and that seems to be a particularly apt metaphor for this book. Daphne Gray-Grant was the first person to help me put pen to paper and nurtured me through the first months. Every pregnancy needs to be greeted with great shouts of joy and those came from Louise Hager and Carol Dale at the bookstore Women In Print. Then, Mike Schwartzentruber was the editor/"midwife" who patiently and gracefully guided the production of the handwritten manuscript into book format. At the time of delivery, Dr. Margaret Merrifield, with overwhelming generosity and enthusiasm, suggested clarifications and wrote the foreword. Words cannot express my gratitude; this book is a labor of love from all of them.

Finally, I would like to acknowledge my husband, Tony Hickling, who not only supported my work, but who is a full partner in our marriage and in our home. Our three children – Margaret, Rob, and J.S. – now adults, did not always enjoy having "the sex lady" as their mother. Only once did they suggest that I take up talking about house repairs instead of sexual health education. Another family member who is always my "helper/teacher" whenever I teach at his school is my grandson, Nicholas Hickling. Thank you to everyone. I am certain that I have missed naming dozens of others, but I thank them all from the bottom of my heart.

What Your Children Need to Know and When They Need to Know It

1

Let's Talk

This class was okay and told me alot of things I never ever new about

I enjoy every single time you come. It's totally worth while. Thanx

I think that this program is important because it can save peoples lives.

I think you should talk more about sex so people will be more awar and more understanding about the topic

Several years ago, in a fifth grade classroom, I was teaching sexual health to a group of 10- and 11-year-olds. When I began to explain that the penis goes into the vagina for the sperm to be delivered to the ovum, the boys began to squirm and talk excitedly to each other.

"Oh yeah, I saw it in a movie, it is so gross! You have to take off all your clothes and lie on top of the girl and hold her really tight."

"Imagine having to do that to a dumb girl!"

Finally, they turned back to me and said, "If only guys had 'stretchable things,' then you wouldn't have to touch her, you could just spray her like a firefighter, to get the baby started!"

That's when I began to think about sexual health education as a "stretchable thing." Many parents had no information given to them by their parents, their churches, or their schools, when they were growing up, and they need to *stretch* their own knowledge and maturity levels to provide it for their children. And the information itself needs to be stretchable, simple to begin, a little and basic in the preschool years, but stretchable as they grow, or when they ask questions, or are exploited.

I rarely meet parents who don't *want* to talk, but I often meet parents who don't know *how* to talk about sexual health. I hope this book will help you to get started and to continue talking and learning.

Naming the Parts – the First Step in Communication

All parents give messages about sexual health from the time their child is born, whether they talk to their child or not. Non-verbal messages through touching, day-to-day child care, facial expressions and actions, all speak volumes to a baby and toddler about sexual health.

It would be helpful if parents could name the genital parts as matter-of-factly as they name elbows. Think for a moment about how we teach babies to talk: "This is your nose; this is your chin; this is your bellybutton..." And then we make a giant leap to the knees!

Or we use baby talk such as "pee-pee," or cutesy names that have been handed down in dad's family for generations and only the Hendersons know what the word means.

We all need to learn vocabulary and to practice using it. When I first began teaching young children, I would say, "Now, I'm going to teach you the polite words for your genital parts; penis is the polite name..." They would all look at me in a puzzled way and say, "Boy, my family must be really rude because we call it a 'dinky' at my house." Or, "My granny must be rude because she calls it a 'ding-dong.'"

I've changed. I now call them scientific words; penis is the scientific name... That lets Granny off the hook; she didn't have these science lessons when she was growing up and she's never had a chance to learn the scientific words.

If you didn't grow up with these names, you need to practice. Say penis 50 times while you are vacuuming and hope your neighbor doesn't call in for coffee while you're doing it!

Begin the day your baby is born by naming the parts. "Now let's wash your

One man phoned me to ask about educating his children – a nine-year-old boy and a ten-year-old girl. He said, "Now understand, Meg, we've taught them some things already. I mean, my daughter has her dickey bird and my son has Mr. Pistol."

Not exactly scientific words!

***

A mother approached me after a family session and, laughing, told me about her very shy husband. When he discovered that she was using the scientific words for the genitals with their four-year-old, he drew her aside and whispered, "If you teach her those words, she'll use them!"

penis, or your vulva." Then by the time your child is old enough to ask, "Why do boys have a penis and girls have a vulva?" you'll feel comfortable.

As the child is able to understand more, you can begin to give him or her more complex information, such as, "The penis is designed to deliver sperm to the ovum to make a baby. It can deliver urine to the toilet too, but you don't have to have a penis to urinate."

Questions and Answers

There are two pieces of old-fashioned and dangerous advice which parents would be well-advised to forget as we move into the 21st century. The first is not to tell a child anything until they ask. "If they're not asking, they're not ready," say the old folks.

Unfortunately, some children will never ask. It doesn't occur to them to be curious in that direction. They ask about rockets, dinosaurs, or Ninjas, but not about bodies and sexual health. For other children, silence on the part of the parents becomes a profound message to the child that this is a taboo subject. "My family does not talk about this, it must be bad, and I'll be in big trouble if I mention 'it,' or ask about 'it.'" Another possibility is that someone else has told them a story – true or untrue – and the child has simply accepted it.

I often meet parents who say, "I want to be the one, or the first one, to tell my child the facts of life." Well, if you want to

A mother said that she had waited all through her son's preschool years for him to ask where babies came from. He never did ask and so she waited all through elementary school. Still no questions. Finally, at age 13, when he was about to enter high school, she decided to have a talk with him. She approached him one evening and said, "I want you to know that I will answer any questions that you might want to ask me, any questions at all."

There was a long silence, and then the boy said, "Well, how do they make glue out of horses?"

be the first, you need not wait for questions – wake them up, tell them, and don't forget to add your moral values and any religious beliefs you have. Children need guidelines and they appreciate reasonable limits.

The second piece of dangerous, old advice is, "Only tell the child what you think they need to know at this time." Parents *always* underestimate what their child "needs" to know. My attempt to maintain a sense of humor includes advising parents to "talk until your child's eyes glaze over."

You cannot tell a child too much; they only take in what they need to know for that moment. This is maddening for some parents. Again they sweat blood. They answer questions fully, thinking, "Thank goodness that is done (for life)!" Two days later they find that the child didn't get it all, or that the child misunderstood what they said and that they have to say it again and again. Keep the doors open, be prepared to talk anytime, and allow, even encourage, the child to come back to a topic over and over.

In an ideal world, one that was truly sexually mature, any adult could answer children's questions with science and health information. But parents often say, "Well, I think that the dads should talk to the boys and the moms to the girls." No way! The best scenario has both parents able to talk to either gender with comfort. There is no reason why dads can't explain menstruation and moms can't explain nocturnal emissions. Single parents especially have to work extra hard at educating themselves about both genders. It is not good enough to say, "I don't know because I am not your gender." Get the books, the videos, the school nurse, or someone else to help you, and share the information together with your child. It is perfectly appropriate to say to your child, "I don't know, but let's find out together."

Grandparents Can Be Teachers Too

Grandparents often tell me that they'd love to talk to their grandchild (they want to do a better job than they did with the child's parents!), and they appear in my parent meetings at elementary schools these days. They tell me that they are providing after-school care for their grandchildren when both parents are at work, or even full care in their own homes.

"Grandma, what is sex?"

"It is whether you're a boy or a girl"

"Oh, I thought it was if you had hair under your arms you were a boy 'cuz girls don't have hair."

Who gets the child's questions after school? Grandma or Grandpa often feel honored that they are hearing the questions, but like parents, they are hesitant about what or how much to say. Several have said that it is difficult to discuss the subject with the child's parents, and yet the grandparent knows that the child will not always get an answer if they use the old, familiar line, "Ask your mother."

I am always delighted to see grandparents who are so committed to their grandchildren's health and safety. In fact, after listening to my presentation, they say, "I've learned so much tonight and I want to ask, where were you when I was growing up?"

I encourage them to answer the questions, to educate themselves *and* those parents, to demonstrate enthusiasm and joy about healthy attitudes throughout the whole extended family. There are wonderful moments in classrooms when children say, "Yes, my grandma talked to me about body science," or "My grandpa read a book about bodies with me." I always want to do a dramatic "thumbs up" and shout, "Yeah, for grandparents!"

Just for fun, here is a book that I recommend for older folks in their personal lives: *Sex May Be Wasted On The Young*, by Lee and Michael Stones (Captus Press, 1996).

Accept the Questions Graciously

Whether you're a parent or a grandparent, try to remember that when children *do* ask questions, no matter how hard the question or how shocking, never be mad! Parents' anger is what children fear most. If you can't think of an answer straight away, tell the child: "I need time to think about this, I promise we will talk about it after supper," or whenever. Please don't cross your fingers and hope that they won't ask again. If the child doesn't ask, bring it up and explain your unease if necessary. "My parents never talked to me, but I'm really proud that you asked me and I'm going to do my best to answer your question."

Bedtime is a great time to talk to young ones because they'll do anything to stop you from leaving and turning out the light. This is a good time to get a book and to start reading to them or to answer questions they may have asked earlier that day on a crowded bus or at Christmas dinner!

One dad told me that his seven-year-old son asked, "What's a blow job?" at the Christmas dinner. This dad responded, "We'll talk about that at bedtime, son." I congratulated him on his wisdom, but he said, "Yeah right, Meg. My biggest problem was all my relatives begging to stay for bedtime too."

You may wish to talk to your child about good manners and/or privacy when giving them detailed information. It is perfectly all right to say, "I am really proud of you for asking this question and I know that you are grown-up enough to have a scientific answer. But perhaps it would not be a good idea to go to school tomorrow and tell everyone what we've talked about. Some parents like to tell their children themselves and their children haven't asked them yet." Or, "Talking about bodies or sexual health embarrasses Granny – she didn't have this science when she was growing up. So is it okay if we don't talk about this on Sunday when Granny comes to dinner?"

Always praise your child for his or her maturity and set out your expectations for good manners. At the same time, don't expect them to always get it right. All of us love to have news to relay, gossip to pass on, and startling new discoveries to share. This kind of thing is the spice of human interaction, for children as well as for adults. Learning about vulvas should be fun as well as fascinating and they may pass on the good news to the cashier in a crowded supermarket. Ignore the smirks, the looks of horror, and the bashful red faces of the others in the grocery line. Be proud that your child is well-educated and protected. If and when we finally drag our whole society into sexual maturity, no one will be upset or think anything of a child's natural curiosity and willingness to share.

Some parents hesitate to tell their children the facts of life in a straightforward, truthful manner for fear that the child will tell the neighbors. My reply to that is, "If the neighbors are hearing the facts of life from a four-year-old for the first time, all you can do is feel sorry that no one has told them the truth before this!" Why would parents want to protect their neighbors and not their

One mother spoke up at a parents' meeting and said, "But, Meg, if I tell my son everything, he'll go to school, tell everybody, and then everyone will know how we got him."

Her friend, who was sitting beside her, began to laugh and said, "Lorraine, it is the same for all of us."

"Oh, I never thought of that," said Lorraine.

child? The only question a parent should ask is, "Did my child tell it correctly?"

Why Your Child Needs To Know This

Some people will say, "I don't think that children need to know about sexuality at this age; I want them to be innocent; I want them to enjoy their childhood."

I like to respond to this concern by pointing out three things.

First, I hear shame in those statements, a reflection of the adult's own childhood where sexuality information was considered to be secret, dirty, for adults only, and smutty. Many of us carry that teaching with us.

But think about it like a scientist. There is nothing shameful about the way we make babies and even less shame in learning about our bodies. We adults need to force ourselves, force our communities, to grow up. We must become more sexually mature to help our children. Granted, it is very difficult to become more mature than our parents were, but our children are depending on us.

Second, knowledge is protection. I don't enjoy visiting prisons, but I do it whenever I am invited because these men can teach me so much about how they exploit, seduce, trick, and trap children into exploitative situations.

Offenders become very skillful at choosing vulnerable children. (Most of them were abused themselves, so they know what to look for.) One thing offenders know is that children do not learn scientific vocabulary from watching *Sesame Street* or any other educational show for children. If a *child* knows appropriate sexual vocabulary, the *offender* knows that some enlightened adult, usually the parent, has taught them. The offender also knows that in the very teaching, the adult has said, "This is an acceptable topic for us to talk about. You are allowed, even encouraged, to know about your body." Because these children know that it's okay to discuss sex with their mom and dad, they are far more likely to tell their parents if someone tries to take advantage of them.

This is why sexually intrusive people will almost always choose a victim who knows nothing and hence, will not tell either. The silence on the part of the parent has become a powerful message not to talk about it.

So please, don't set your child up to be vulnerable. An innocent or uneducated child is unsafe and poorly protected.

(I do, by the way, have some sympathy for the abuser. This is not to excuse the abuse, but sometimes the stories of their own childhood abuse are enough to make you weep. And abusers often say, "If only I had had the education that you provide, Meg, when I was a kid, I might not be sitting in jail now with this trail of destruction behind me.")

Third, when we teach children about conception and how it happens through sexual intercourse, we are not teaching them to have sex. Nor are we saying that it would be appropriate for them to have sex. Intercourse is an adult activity. As I've said, many children are very glad to hear that and will say, "I am never doing that."

What we are teaching children is "body science." They may never have sexual intercourse, but they will always have bodies to care for, and sexual health is no different than nutritional health.

Disabled Children

Parents of children with disabilities need to be especially proactive about providing sexual health education to their children, even in the preschool and primary years. Disabled children have the same right to be informed and they have an even greater need for the protection that this information provides. Research indicates that disabled children suffer up to five times more abuse than other children and youth.

Children with physical or intellectual challenges are often at greater risk of abuse or sexual exploitation as teens or young adults because they are more isolated in the community, and because they are often taught to be passive and obedient, and to trust all caregivers.

They may lack the boundaries, communication skills, and social skills which could help to keep them safe.

Although we often think of disabled children as asexual, this simply isn't true. They are sexual beings, just like everybody else. Disabled children usually go through puberty at exactly the same time as other children do and they have similar worries and concerns about body changes.

The challenge for parents and caregivers is that the health and safety concepts about sexual health need to be given again and again, with patience, humor, and compassion. Fortunately, there are wonderful resources available to help parents teach disabled children. Don't hesitate to call your local health facility for help. You may also encourage your local parent association to be actively involved in making resources available.

And remember, there's lots of fun to be had teaching children with disablilities – as this story illustrates so well: In a class of physically and mentally disabled teens, several boys told me that a famous porn star had died the day before. As I began to talk about AIDS in the pornography industry, one of the girls said, "Oh, I saw him in a magazine. He had a very long penis." Another girl, who had been silent all morning, suddenly spoke and said, "He probably tripped over it and killed himself." It brought the house down, as they say.

What Your Children Need to Know and When They Need to Know It

Of course, children don't mature all at once and so their education doesn't have to happen all at once.

Researchers have studied the sexual development of children from around the world, from many different countries, from all sorts of families, ethnic groups, economic and educational levels. Their findings are fascinating, but most parents have neither the time nor the inclination to read their massive volumes.

When I began teaching in the mid-1970s, I read their work and revised their theories of stage development to mimic the stages of education that children go through in the public schools.

After 20 years of honing my own observations and experience with children of all ages, their parents, and the professionals who work with children in medicine, education, theology and social sciences, I see the "stages" more as pads in a lily pond. We all spend time on the various pads at different points, depending on the situation, our own education, experience, and maturity.

Imagine a lily pond with "nirvana," the sexually mature adult island, in the middle. The ideal situation would be to spend as much time there as possible. Near the shore, there are the preschoolers' pads. Out a bit, but not far, are the primary pads. In the middle are the intermediate pads. And closer to the sexually mature island are the adolescent pads.

Each pad has wonderful flowers that we can pick and take with us, but there are also thorns that can get stuck in us and cause discomfort, pain, and even life-threatening illnesses.

Sometimes, through lack of education or positive life experience, people get stuck on one pad for a long time, or forever. Some people continually hop back and forth, never coming close to or reaching nirvana. And some are kept, by forces beyond themselves, on one or two pads.

In the next four chapters, I will be writing about the stages of sexual development that children and teens go through in most countries today. But in countries such as Sweden, Holland, and Protestant Germany, where sexual health education has been mandatory in the schools for several generations, children do not go through the magical thinking of the preschoolers, the bathroom humor of the primaries, or the "gross-me-outs" of the intermediates with anything like the intensity that children from other countries do.

Today, parents in Sweden, for instance, were brought up by parents who were well-educated and sexually mature themselves, who talked openly and factually about sexuality and sexual health, and who carried little of the emotional baggage and repression that others have around the issues of sexual health. The statistical evidence of health is there to see: lower rates of sexual abuse, sexual exploitation, abortion, suicide, teenage pregnancy, and STDs (sexually transmitted diseases). Perhaps, one day, we will learn by their example, and progress to new and brighter islands of sexual maturity.

A "Triple-whammy"

It seems to me that parents today have a "triple-whammy." Most want to talk to their children more honestly than their parents did. (So do many grandparents!) So the first task is to educate ourselves with all the new information. The second task is to be more comfortable and to pass it on to our children. And the third task is to recognize that you are educating others in the family and community as well.

Here's a funny story which is also a great example of how everyone in the family and community could benefit from further education.

One mother of a preschool age daughter said that she had heard that you should tell children that boys have a penis and girls have a vulva.

So she taught her daughter that she had a vulva. Like all three-year-olds, the daughter was keen to share the news.

Not long after, grandmother arrived from Montreal for Christmas. An hour after Granny's arrival, the little girl asked, "Granny, do you have a vulva?"

"No, dear," said Granny, "I have a Toyota."

2

Preschoolers
Magical Thinkers
(Ages Two – Four)

---

how do you make baby's

Do women always have flaps on their virgina.

Can people urinate while they have sex?

How is a bayby born?.

My brother was born with only one testicle. would it effect his sperm

Parents who have been sheltered themselves, or who grew up in repressed homes, often ask, "Why do I have to talk to my child now, at his age? She doesn't ask questions; he's not interested; she will be shocked; he will be upset; she will look at me (us) differently; I want to keep him innocent; I want them to have their childhood; they don't need to know now..."

As I indicated in the previous chapter, I think all of this is actually saying, "I am not ready, I don't know what to say, I am still embarrassed," and most of all, "I was upset when I found out and I don't want my child to go through the horrors I went through."

I need to repeat myself here because this is just so important. There are three reasons for beginning to talk with children in the preschool years and all of them have to do with prevention.

1. Children in the preschool years are the easiest to talk with. They accept the information like sponges. You are teaching them science and health. Don't let your silence teach your child that your family cannot talk about this subject.

2. Children need years to understand and absorb the information that you want to give them – your family values, morality, and theology. Don't allow someone else or the media to do it for you with myths, misunderstandings, deviancy, and exploitation.

Two moms, one obviously very pregnant, told me with gales of laughter about their two preschoolers: Eric, who is expecting a sibling soon; and Todd, who knows nothing about babies, but lots about geography.

Eric: Todd, do you know that babies come from vaginas?

Todd: They don't come from China.

Eric: No, not China, they come from down there.

Todd: Down there is Australia and I don't think they come from Australia, either.

3. Studies from all over the world consistently show that children who are educated about healthy bodies and healthy sexuality are protected from abuse and exploitation. Children need vocabulary and information to protect themselves against sexual abuse. If you wait for children to ask questions before giving this information, you may wait forever.

Besides providing these preventatives for your young children, early childhood sexual health education pays off when they get older as well. Teens and young adults who have learned in an open way at home are far less sexually active, promiscuous, and unsafe in relationships. They also feel more secure, happy, and successful in their daily lives.

Magical Thinking

When preschoolers don't have factual information about something, they make up a story to explain things to themselves. Educational psychologists call this "magical thinking." An example of dangerous magical thinking is what happens when some boys know nothing about urination. They imagine that their urine comes from their testicles and then, when they are in a hurry to urinate, they stand at the toilet and squeeze their testicles to make the urine come out faster. Testicles can be damaged and there isn't a lot of sensitivity there until puberty begins. Have you ever noticed how preschool boys can grab their genitals and haul them up to their navels? Their dads are yelping with sympathetic pain; the little ones don't feel it, but damage can occur.

Preschoolers also do a lot of magical thinking around the issues of reproduction, if no one tells them the truth. Some decide that if you want a baby, you go to the hospital. The hospital, they imagine, has rooms full of babies and the nurses hand them out to anyone who asks for one.

One mother courageously confessed that she'd found herself stuck at this stage. She told her elder child that she was going to the hospital to get a baby and he said he'd like a boy baby, not a girl baby. She said, "I'll see what I can do." When she brought home a baby girl, he said, "I don't want a baby sister, take it back and change it." She told him that the hospital was all out of boy babies and they had to take this one.

Stork stories, cabbage patches, and foundlings are all examples of adults doing magical thinking because they are not mature enough themselves to tell the truth.

When the parent is honest and says that the penis goes into the vagina to deliver the sperm to the ovum, most preschoolers will say, "Oh. Can we have lunch now?" The parent may sweat blood, but the child is fine.

The only challenge at this stage is to be prepared to tell the story again and again. Preschoolers don't always understand it fully the first time, or they only take in a bit of what was said, or more commonly, some other person comes along with a better story and if mom and/or dad is not able to continue talking, they choose to believe the last person who talked.

Preschoolers are the easiest of all children to teach about sexual health. They carry no emotional baggage. (We adults carry tons of emotional baggage. We didn't have parents who talked openly with us – girls may have got some menses education at school, boys usually got nothing, and we all grew up in a sexually repressed

---

One mom told me how much she and her five-year-old daughter had enjoyed a recently published book called *What's the Big Secret?* about sexuality and reproduction, written by Laurie and Marc Brown.

She then overheard her daughter telling a friend, "Max, boys can't have babies."

"I know that," said Max.

"Yes, but do you know why not?" she asked. "Because boys don't have room and no pajamas!"

society.) The best thing about this age is that preschoolers have loads of intellectual curiosity. They accept information about their bodies in the same matter-of-fact way they accept information about anything else, so why not share it?

Boys' Bodies

The penis, then, is designed for its real job – delivering sperm. The penis can only deliver sperm when it is erect and so boys' penises begin to practice erections 17 weeks into the pregnancy. Practice erections happen many times each day. Daytime erections are not as vigorous after puberty, but all healthy males have several erections while they are asleep.

An erection does not mean that your child has to go to the bathroom; he may have a full bladder when he wakes up, but that is a coincidence. Think about it like a scientist. When the penis gets erect, there is a valve at the mouth of the bladder which closes tightly so that no urine can escape. It allows free passage of sperm through the urethra without contamination by urine. Nature would not send a signal that you have to go to the bathroom and then turn off the water works!

Erections are often simply practice erections. I call them "push-up exercises to keep your penis healthy." Boys and girls need to be reassured about spontaneous

A three-year-old boy, when I said that the father's penis delivers the sperm to the mother's ovum:

"Yeah," he shouted gleefully, "and my father plants radishes too!"

What if you have to pee durring Set?

Why does a penis erect?

A mom told me about her preschool son, who had never been able to fully retract his foreskin, as many young boys can't. One day he had been sitting in the bath for a very long time – long enough for the foreskin to soften enough so that he could retract it. He came rushing out of the bathroom with an enormous erection, foreskin pulled back, and said, "Mom, look! I've got TWO!!"

Mom, at a total loss for words, said, "Go show your father."

***

Another mum told me about the first time her preschool son saw a circumcised penis at the local swimming pool. Her son came running up to her and said, "Mum, come quick! Scotty's penis is falling out!"

erections, otherwise the silence or the embarrassed reaction from parents and others becomes a message of guilt, shame, and taboo.

Talk to your son about his penis – how it works, how to take care of it (wash it like a finger, he may not be able to fully retract or pull back the foreskin until he goes into puberty) and help him to feel comfortable so that if he gets an infection or an injury he will be able to tell you right away without shame.

It's also a good idea to be able to explain circumcision, because young children see both circumcised and uncircumcised penises, often when they go swimming and change out of their bathing suits.

Here's what I say to children who have questions: All baby boys are born with loose, movable skin at the end of their penis; it's called foreskin. Sometimes, the doctor or a special religious person removes the foreskin. This is called circumcision. If you have your penis circumcised, it still works exactly the same way as an uncircumcised penis, so it's not anything to worry about.

In the old days, almost all baby boys in North America were circumcised because we thought it would help them to stay clean and healthy. Nowadays, we know that soap and water is enough to keep penises clean and healthy, so we no longer circumcise every baby boy. It really is left up to the parents to decide. Parents from the Jewish religion and the Muslim religion believe in circumcision for religious reasons, and so their sons are always circumcised.

Remember that girls need to know too. This is science and health information.

Usually, boys are born with two testicles in the scrotum or scrotal sac behind the penis, between their legs. (You can be perfectly healthy and fertile with only one testicle.)

Naturally, many boys call them balls because of their shape. (It is fun, and scientific, to point out that girls have balls too. Theirs are called ovaries and are inside the girl's body, one on either side of the uterus. They are left inside her body because the ova – "eggs" in slang language – need to be kept warm.) Testicles and ovaries are also known by another scientific name: gonads.

Boys' testicles are moved from inside to outside the body at birth because they have to be kept cooler: four to five degrees cooler than body temperature. The scrotum is made of special skin that is stretchable and shrinkable, so that the testicles can be pulled closer to keep them warm, or allowed to move away from the body to keep them cool.

That is also why, once toilet training is completed, it is not healthy for your child to wear tight underwear to bed every night. As I explain to children, "You'll make your testicles too hot. That is also why they make

If a boy has only one testacle will he produce enough testosterone and sperm to be "normal"?

pajamas with a deep crotch, so there's room for air conditioning at night. Or you could just sleep in a T-shirt, or nude!"

I love it when kids tell me that their dad sleeps nude. "Great," I say. "Your dad has the healthiest testicles in the world." The dads and moms usually roar with joy at this response. The kids, however, still aren't sure. "What if there is a fire?" they ask. I reassure them by saying, "Take your sheet, but don't forget that your life is worth more than your nudity, so go naked if you have to and don't worry. All fire trucks have blankets. The firefighters will give you one. They *hate* fighting fires with naked people watching!"

The testicles make two things: sperm, "So that you can be a father when you grow up (if you want to be)"; and more important to boys, testosterone, a growth hormone. "That is pretty important, so take good care of them. Don't kick or punch or squeeze anyone's testicles. And keep them cool."

Sometimes preschoolers listen to all the information and then they say, "Yes, and you know what? You should never let anyone step on your testicles either." I think that that is good advice.

When messages of health and science are given in this way, boys will feel comfortable telling parents when and if they have problems.

One potential problem parents should be aware of occurs when the blood supply to the testicles – and ovaries too – gets twisted. This is called a "torsion." If this happens, immediate emergency intervention is necessary.

In a kindergarten class:
Meg: Now, try to think like a scientist. Why did nature put the boys' testicles on the outside?

Kids: To keep them cool.

Meg: Okay. Now why are the girls' ovaries on the inside?

Little girl: Because we're prettier?

In boys of all ages, a torsion can be caused by a hit, but it can also happen even when there is no obvious reason. If your son complains of testicular pain or swelling, don't wait around. Go to a doctor immediately.

Although twisting of the blood supply to the ovaries is rarer, it is important to recognize the possibility. If your daughter, no matter how young (even a three-year-old) complains of intermittent, intense abdominal pain, nausea, vomiting, fever, or loss of appetite, ask your doctor about a sonogram.

Sometimes parents feel shy about testicular pain and hesitate to take their child to a hospital or clinic. Sometimes the child is so shy they will resist examination. And believe it or not, sometimes *doctors* hesitate because of shyness, or because of lack of experience with torsions. Some doctors might simply give antibiotics, hoping that the pain and fever are simply caused by an infection. It never hurts to ask, "Could we rule out an ovarian or testicular torsion?"

Boys have two openings between their legs. One opening is the urethra, at the end of the penis, where the urine and sperm come out. It is important to explain that everyone's bladder collects urine and is in the same place, just under the skin, above the pubic bone. Both boys and girls have a urethra, the tube that drains the bladder: girls have a short urethra and so they sit down to urinate; boys have a longer urethra, so they may stand to urinate.

The other opening is the anus, where the stool comes out. Use stool as the scientific word – among several that could be used – because doctors ask for stool samples. (You'd look funny bringing your doctor your piano stool.)

A mother told her son that the word "Willy" was his dad's nickname for the penis. "But the scientific name is penis," she said.

The little boy thought for a moment, and then, pointing to his backside, said, "Oh, so is this my poo-nis?"

It is perfectly appropriate to get a hand mirror and let children have a look between their legs so that they can "be scientists" and know about their bodies. A natural time for this healthy exploration is during bath time, when parents are present to supervise and make certain exploitation of a sibling does not occur.

Whoever says "no," rules. If one child does not want to be explored, that child rules. Parents should be within earshot at bath time, if not actually present, to protect each child's privacy.

Girls' Bodies

"Boys have two openings in their genitals. How many do girls have between their legs?"

Almost always, children in my classes say, "One."

We, as adults, set them up with this misinformation when we tell children that boys have a penis and girls have a vagina. Children then believe that girls have one giant opening between their legs and that everything comes out of it, or they believe that vagina is the name for everything between the female legs. It is much better to say, "Boys have a penis and girls have a vulva."

Vulva is the name for the outside skin on a girl's genitals. It is folded skin. The scientific name for these folds is labia.

Smegma is the name for the white cheesy secretions that form between the folds of the vulva and under the skin of the foreskin on the penis. Smegma is produced for cleansing and lubrication, it is normal and healthy, nothing to be ashamed about. Children simply need to be taught to wash it away, just like washing behind their ears.

At the front of the girl's vulva, where the folds come together, is a part of the

What is the clitoris there for

body called the clitoris. The visible part of the clitoris is as big as the end of your baby finger and it can become erect when she is sexually excited. However, the clitoris doesn't "practice" erections like the penis does. The "tickling" feeling that girls sometimes report is due to extra blood moving into the genital area during sexual arousal. Vaginal moisture may also increase during arousal.

This is perhaps a good time to acknowledge that all children are born with the ability to have an orgasm, and genital feelings of sexual arousal may occur in children at a very young age. Children who are not educated about these very normal responses can feel shame and guilt.

Given healthy, accepting messages, children will often report erections and "tingly vaginas" when watching sexual images on television. One two-year-old watching a bedroom scene on a soap opera said, "Mummy, when those people do that my vagina tickles." A good response would be something like this: "Yes, that is normal. It will stop in a minute."

Not that I want this to happen, but it happens to me and I want to know what it is. Every once in a while my crotch feels like it is being tickled. (I'm a girl)

Adults also need to remind children that although the feelings are normal and healthy, they are also private. It is not polite to tell others who may not want to hear about your sexual excitement. Mom and Dad are fine, but perhaps not Granny, or the babysitter, or the visitor. This is another example of good manners, health, and privacy.

Moving on, just behind the clitoris is the urethra, where the urine comes out. Behind that is the vagina, where the baby comes out.

The vagina is about as long as your middle finger and it stretches open by 10 centimeters to let out the baby. The best science for your child to know about the vagina is that as soon as the baby comes out, the vagina closes again. Women are not walking around with huge black holes between their legs.

This is how I talk about the vagina with young children: The vagina is the cleanest opening in the whole human body. It constantly makes moisture, just like your eyes do. Sometimes the moisture comes out of the vagina during the day and you can see it on the toilet paper; it looks like water during most of the month and like raw egg white when the ovum (egg) is released from the ovary. This is the time of month when you are most likely to get pregnant. Sometimes it dries to a yellowish or whitish color on your underpants. That is a good sign that your vagina is clean and healthy.

The vagina is the opening for the baby to come out but also for the penis to enter to deliver the sperm. When the woman is pleased to be having sexual intercourse, her vagina actually opens a little to accept the penis and it makes extra moisture to make it slippery and not painful.

When a woman is very nervous about having sex, or feeling ashamed or guilty, the vagina may not make extra moisture or open. In this case, sex can be painful. If someone forces her to have sex (that is called rape or sexual assault) the skin and inside tissue can be torn and it can be very painful.

Again, whoever says "no," rules. Sexual intercourse is for adults and even

---

One mom had begun to teach her son the scientific names but recognized that there was still work to do when he told his grandmother that "the father delivers his sperm to the mother's 'cajoiner.'"

***

A mom told me that her husband came in from collecting their five-year-old from day care and asked, "Why is Shawn learning about ladies' china at school?"

when you are an adult, you do not have to have sex if you don't want to. In fact, you never have to have sex in your whole life if you don't want to.

At this point, many children will say, "Good, I'm never having sex." Parents can reply, "But you still have to learn about your body and how to take care of it. You will always have sexual health to be concerned about, whether you are sexually active or not."

Finally, behind the vagina, is the anus where the stool comes out.

Where Babies Come From

This is how I describe it to children in a class about body science: Once the sperm has been delivered to the ovum, a baby begins to grow. The baby grows in the uterus, a special bag made of strong muscle, behind the bladder, in the bottom of the pelvis or abdomen. It sits on top of the vagina and is about as big as your four curled fingers.

The uterus stretches bigger and bigger when it has a baby growing in it. It stretches bigger in front of the woman. It is rude and unfair to call a pregnant woman fat. She is not fat; she is stretched. A baby cannot grow inside the abdomen because that part of your body is filled with intestines.

how dose sex make babys

When the baby is born, the uterus goes smaller again, just like letting air out of a balloon.

The baby actually grows in two bags: the outer one, made of muscle, is called the uterus; the inner one is filled with water. Nature provides the water (or amniotic fluid) as protection for the baby. If the mother falls down or is in an accident, the baby bounces in the water and remains safe.

Of course, if the baby is underwater it cannot breathe or eat, so it grows an umbilical cord from the bellybutton (or navel) which is wide open out to the wall of the uterus. The blood vessels in the cord bring the baby oxygen, vitamins, and nutrients from the mother's blood. The baby doesn't get real food, like chips and peas; its stomach is not working. It is a good thing that the baby doesn't get real food – otherwise it would go poo in there and that would be messy!

When it is time for the baby to be born, the strong muscles of the uterus begin to squeeze and relax, squeeze and relax. This is called contractions. The contractions usually go on for several hours.

At this point, I love pointing out to the children that the baby loves the contractions. They feel like giant hugs and actually prepare the baby to breathe. It is really helpful for the baby to experience labor. (By this time, I have parents with tears in their eyes, listening to this story. Many women have said, "If only I'd known that when I was in labor!")

A mother and her young daughter were at the swimming pool when they saw a woman with five or six young children. The little girl asked her mom to help her count the children. When they counted six, the child sighed and said, "Boy, she sure must have a tired vagina."

After several hours, the squeezing pops the water bag and the water comes out of the vagina, making it wet and slippery, just like a waterslide. So the very first waterslide that you ever had was when you came slip sliding out of your mom's vagina. It is great fun for the baby and hard, hard work for the mom.

Sometimes the mother cannot push her baby out of her vagina and then the doctor has to make a cut in the mother's uterus and take the baby out that way. This is called being born by Cesarean or C-section.

Often, someone asks, "Why does the baby come out crying?" The answer is that babies *don't* necessarily come out crying. Some do because the lights are so bright, or because it is cold. But lots of babies come out smiling, even humming a little song to themselves. We no longer hold babies up by their heels – that can damage their spinal cords – and we no longer smack them. We don't want them to cry. A newborn needs to breathe deeply and calmly, so that's why we put them straight onto their mom's chest to be cuddled.

When the baby is breathing properly, the doctor or midwife can cut the cord near the baby's bellybutton with very clean scissors. This is just like cutting your hair; it doesn't hurt the mother or the baby. A few days later, the little bit of cord that was left dries up and falls off. Meanwhile, your bellybutton (or umbilicus or navel) has closed itself in a scar and it will never come open again. It is your very first scar. Some people have "innie" scars and some have "outie" scars; no one knows exactly why.

A few minutes after the baby is born, when the uterus begins to shrink, the mother helps to push out the other end of the umbilical cord. Some children think that the doctor pushes it back in for the next baby, but each baby grows its own cord.

Who Would Believe *That?*

Here is a true story that confirms both the wisdom of providing sexual health information as a means of preventing abuse, and the reality of a young child's ability to appreciate "the facts of life."

A parent of a preschooler told me that she had years of experience as a prosecutor of sexual offenders and she had never met a child victim who had been educated about sexual health. Instinctively, when her son was born, she and her husband taught him the scientific names for genitals plus the facts of reproduction. When he was five, he watched a movie with his parents that depicted storks bringing animal and human babies. He was very curious: "What is *that* all about?" he asked.

His parents explained that in the old days parents told children that storks brought babies. He stared at them with amazement and then said, "Who would believe *that*?"

Who indeed?

Explaining Menses to Young Children

It is always a good idea to be able to explain menstruation, or periods, to young children – boys as well as girls.

I explain periods this way: When a girl's body begins to grow and practice for being grown-up, her uterus practices too. Some girls begin to practice when they are eight or nine years old, others some time after that.

The uterus practices by making a kind of "water bed" inside itself for the baby. It is made of water, soft skin, and a little bit of blood. Each month, when there isn't a baby there, the uterus changes the bed and the old one comes dripping out of the vagina.

It looks like drops of blood, but it is mostly water. It is clean and healthy and it is called "having your period." The scientific word is "menstruation."

You have to wear a pad in your pants to catch the drips. The ads for these on television are really silly. On television, the pads soak up blue water and they have wings and can fly! In real life, you stick the pad inside your underpants and it sits beside your vagina and catches all the drips. Some women use tampons which are inserted in the vagina (the string hangs outside) to absorb the drips from inside.

Why do they use blue water

What are those thing with wings on T.V.?

We are really glad that girls and women have periods. It is your body practicing for having a baby.

When discussing tampons, remind them that the vagina is only as deep as your middle finger, it can't get lost in there and the string will not break. You may also want to explain that the tampons have special additives added to the cotton, so that they won't leak. I tell children that a few women still get a bacterial infection called toxic shock syndrome, so you may choose not to wear tampons. Some children are horrified by tampons and I like to respond by saying that, "You never have to wear tampons if you don't want to, you can always use pads. It is a personal choice."

Some women are quite comfortable having their youngsters in the bathroom with them when they are menstruating, and comfortable talking to them about sanitary products. Other mothers need more privacy and don't feel comfortable. There is no "right" way to be, except to be open to talking to them about menstruation as a clean and healthy process.

You may have trouble imagining yourself having this kind of conversation with your young child, but believe me, it's worth it. And here's the proof.

One mother told me that she had dragged her husband to the preschool meeting to hear me. He was clearly uncomfortable and stared at me as if I was from Mars, all through the presentation. He said very little to her on the way home, but did say that he had learned a few things, and since they had two daughters, perhaps it was good to have been there.

She said that several weeks later, their two preschool-age girls came bounding into their bed as usual in the morning. The mother discovered that her period had started in the night and she quickly left for the bathroom, which was located off the bedroom. The girls noticed the stain on the sheet and asked, with some alarm, what had happened.

The mother could hear her husband plump the pillows up against the headboard and begin to tell them about menstruation, "using all your words, Meg, and doing a beautiful job. He made it sound natural, clean, and healthy. He even told them that when they began to have periods, he'd be so proud 'because your bodies will be practicing for being grown-up.'"

It still brings tears to my eyes when I think about that wonderful father, forcing himself to be calm, mature, and delighting in his task as educator for his daughters. And now the best part: according to the mother, the girls listened attentively, asked a few questions, then shrugged their shoulders and said, "Okay. Now, Dad, can we have some scrambled eggs for breakfast?"

Wet Dreams and Testicles

Don't forget to explain that boys' bodies practice for being grown-up, too. They get "wet dreams." The scientific name is "nocturnal emissions," or "sperm that come out at night!"

I like to explain wet dreams this way: When boys are eight or nine years old, or older, their testicles begin to make sperm for practice. Some nights, when boys are fast asleep, the extra sperm come out of his penis. Only one spoonful of milky-white fluid comes out and it makes a small wet spot on his pajamas or between his legs. It is clean and healthy and we're glad that boys' bodies practice for being grown-up, too.

I like to point out to parents and to children that menstruation and nocturnal emissions are normal, healthy functions. They are *private*, of course, but they are not a *secret*. Everyone knows about these functions and when we learn about them we are learning about science and health.

Condom Caution

I have talked for over 30 years to preschoolers and school-age children about condoms simply because their parents begged me to talk about them. Children find condoms all over the place – in parks, at the beach, on the streets, and in schoolyards. Many parents were raised with negative messages about condoms: only prostitutes use them, they are filthy, they are for diseased men... I have seen parents' faces wrinkle in disgust when I bring condoms out of my teaching kit.

I prefer to start my condom talk on a positive note. "Condoms are clean and healthy when you buy them. They are made of the same rubber (latex) as a doctor's rubber gloves." I always use a good quality condom, not a colored or joke condom. I put the condom over my two fingers and then I continue: "When two grownups love each other a lot, they love to have sex a lot." Predictably, groans and "oohs" emerge from the children and I use that moment to say, "If your parents still have sex, you are very lucky because that means that they love each other a lot." Happy smiles often break out on the children's faces following this simple statement, because most kids know their parents have sex but have never had any positive statement about it.

Then I continue: "But, although parents might have sex until they die, they may not want to have 35 babies." There will be great choruses of agreement and understanding from the kids at this point. "So, the man puts the condom over his penis and then, when his penis goes into her vagina and the sperm come out, they get caught in the condom and don't go into her body to make a baby." Huge sighs of relief emerge from the children and a look of sudden enlightenment appears on their faces.

What's a condom

Now comes the caution: "When polite people have finished having sex, they take the condom off and put it in their own private garbage at home. But sometimes, people are rude and they throw condoms out in parks and at schools and at the beach where children can find them – and the condoms do not always look like this one. Sometimes they are different colors and sometimes they have pictures on them.

"They look like balloons, but you must not pick them up. Go and tell an adult. It is not your job to pick up condoms and put them in the garbage."

I've also begun to show the children the new female condoms because they are now appearing on the streets. One boy said, "Oh man, I'm glad you told me what that was, because I would have taken it home and kept my marbles in it." They *do* look like cool "baggies."

Although there have been no reported cases of children becoming sick from handling a used condom, we are particularly concerned about the hepatitis viruses which may survive for a long time in dried human fluid. So many children report that they have found condoms and have then tried to blow them up or make water bombs out of them.

Finally, I like to return to the positive message about condoms. "Condoms are like tissue. They are very clean and healthy when you buy them at the store, they help to keep germs from spreading from one person to another, but you wouldn't pick up a tissue that you found outside, so don't pick up condoms either."

One mom told me about waiting at a bus stop with her five-year-old and ten-year-old sons, when the younger boy spotted a condom. The mother said that her heart nearly stopped with panic as she pulled him away because she didn't know what to say. Ten-year-old son to the rescue!

"Don't touch those, Tyler. Men use them to have sex and they can have serious germs on them."

The five-year-old said, "Okay. Can I look at your comic now?"

The mom, filled with gratitude and admiration, asked her son later how he knew that.

"Oh, we learned about that at school in body-science," he said, very matter-of-factly and unembarrassed.

Preschool Checklist

Your preschool child needs to know (before they begin attending school)

- the names for genitals – penis, testicles, scrotum, anus, vulva, labia, vagina, clitoris, uterus, ovaries;
- that reproduction happens when a man's sperm joins a woman's ovum by sexual intercourse;
- that the baby grows in the uterus;
- that the baby is born through the vagina;
- the basics about menses and nocturnal emissions as clean and healthy processes;
- not to pick up condoms.

3

Primaries
The Bathroom Humor Types
(First Grade – Third Grade)

How do you
know which
opening...
put the
Tampon in

How does a man's
penis go into a
ladies virgina?

Why Does gas
smell?

How do you breathe
when you kiss?

In the primary grades, children's favorite jokes center around underwear and bare bums. They can make every word in the English language rhyme with pee, poo, and diarrhea. They are fascinated by elimination and especially by diarrhea. Their favorite thing to do is to fart.

If you think for a moment, you can probably name several friends of yours, even relatives, who are stuck at this level. (Mostly males, dare I say?)

I think that children go through this stage of being mesmerized by elimination because they have the digestive system confused with the reproductive system. That gives elimination an enormous amount of power. All that giggling, exchanging jokes, rhyming, and constant anal attention is a means of exploring and trying to find out about sexuality and sexual health.

We, as immature adults, add to the confusion of our children when we tell them that babies grow in stomachs or tummies, and when we say that boys have a penis and girls have a vagina. We also say that the woman has eggs and the man has seeds – all related to food and digestion. Naturally, children assume from all of this that the woman eats or swallows something to get the baby into her stomach and many imagine that she will "poo" the baby out, or vomit or cough the baby up, or her bellybutton comes open. (So why do boys have bellybuttons?)

In a Primary Family Session:

I get to the part where I say "and the father puts his penis in the mother's vagina for the sperm to be delivered..."

One five-year-old cherub speaks: "Oh my goodness, when I get married I am going to have to tell my wife about this and she is going to be very surprised!"

"Well maybe she will know this already."

"Oh no she won't and she's going to be very embarrassed."

"But perhaps she will have had a science lesson like this."

"Oh no, not my wife, I doubt it."

"Well maybe she is here tonight."

Child takes a quick look around and says, "Nah, I wouldn't marry any of these girls."

I am always amazed by adults who would rather tell children that the doctor cuts open the woman to get the baby out than tell them about a vaginal birth. (By the way, if you had your child by Cesarean, it is fine and good to say that, but please don't pretend that that is how *all* babies are born.)

Let's be fair to those parents who have done a wonderful job of being open and honest with their preschoolers and primaries but who still find them rolling on the floor with their friends in bathroom humor. You didn't give birth to stupid children; they know what they have to do to be part of a peer group, and this is peer pressure.

A study I saw a few years ago suggested that only 30 percent of parents talk with their children at home about sexual health throughout their child's growing years. Imagine how few talk at the preschool age. So your child is at school with the majority of his or her peers who know nothing and who use bathroom humor to explore the subject. In her saner moments, your well-educated child may ask, "Why does Billy always make jokes about dinkys and regina?" Or a more mature child will ask, "Why did everyone laugh about beaver on the television show?" Many adults are stuck at this level and cannot talk about any aspect of sexual health without making it into a big joke. There are days when our whole society seems stuck at this level. Remember AIDS jokes, Bobbitt jokes, and condom jokes?

Finally, remember that the stages are shrinkable and stretchable. If you have a preschooler and a primary, the six-year-old

---

In one primary class, I was explaining vaginal deliveries and said, "The water bag breaks and makes the vagina like a waterslide."

One young fellow said, "Oh no, not me. I wasn't born like that."

Another boy spoke up: "Yes you were, George. My father delivered you!"

has probably dragged your four-year-old into the bathroom humor ahead of time. Or if your well-educated four-year-old only associates with sexually mature adults, she may skip the primary bathroom humor altogether.

Mechanical Curiosity

The wonderful characteristic that primaries have in abundance, and that we wish they could hold on to for all of their lives, is mechanical curiosity. This is the ability to ask without shame or hesitation, "Exactly how does it work?"

Let me illustrate how beautifully they accept the mechanical details.

One mother told me about her joy that I had arrived to teach the children since she had never said one word to her six-year-old son about sexual health.

As they were walking home, she said, "Wasn't that a great lesson about body science?"

The son replied, "Yes, it was fun. But some of it was in French, right Mom?"

***

Six-year-old boy, talking with his dad after a body-science lesson.

"Dad, try to be a scientist and tell me how you get your penis off to deliver the sperm to the lady's vagina?"

I was teaching a large group of primary students in front of all their parents one evening and I arrived at the part where I say, "and the man's penis goes into the woman's vagina to deliver the sperm to her ovum." A little six-year-old girl shot up her hand before I could say another word.

"Wait a minute, wait a minute," she said. "Just where would people do that?"

She calmly waited for the parents to still their laughter and went on. "I mean, would you do that in your house, or would you go to the hospital?"

I could tell from the inflection in her voice that she fully expected me to say, "You go to the hospital and the doctors and nurses supervise this activity." So, since I am always emphasizing to the students that this is a science lesson about bodies, I said, "Oh, probably most people would do this in their own homes, in their beds, at night."

"Oh," she said, obviously accepting the mechanical details.

But her little friend sitting beside her then spoke up, and in a thoughtful, musing way said, "In their beds, at night... I never knew that."

Then she crossed her arms, looked up at me, and said, "Now, what next?" perfectly prepared to go on to the next piece of information that I might have for her.

It was a classical illustration of primary-stage inquiry. Here's another.

When you say to a primary, "The penis goes into the vagina to deliver the sperm to the ovum," a frequent response from a five- or six-year-old would be, "Oh, how long does he leave it in for." Immature adults might be embarrassed or evasive. Mature parents would reply factually and calmly, "Sometimes it only takes a second and sometimes a few minutes." Many children hear family gossip that indicates Uncle Sid and Auntie Alice took five years to have a baby.

It might be funny or cute when six-year-old Suzy thinks that Aunty and Uncle were joined together for five years, but it is not cute when Suzy is 15 and pregnant and she says, "I can't be pregnant, we only did it once, or on Saturdays, or for a year."

It would be wonderful if children could hang on to this quest for details for the rest of their lives. Parents and educators need to welcome the questions and rejoice in

Do people lie down to have sex?

***

In a first grade classroom:
Meg: You were only as big as a grain of sand when you first began.

Child (shouting): Not me. I weighed 10 pounds and my brother was 11.

***

how long does the penis have to stay in the vigina for?

How many times do you have to have sex to have a baby

the mechanical details; they provide golden teachable moments. Treat every question with respect and seize every moment that comes along to give science and health information.

Perhaps most important of all is to never lose your sense of humor. Enjoy the questions, the funny misuse of words, the mispronunciations, the misunderstandings – your own as well as your child's. Children hate to be laughed at and most of all hate to be teased, but our shared laughter is a gift.

The Sensuous Child

Some children are born more sensual than others. The sensual ones adore being cuddled and want a lot of it. They may show a lot of interest in breasts and genitals – their own and yours! If you are not a particularly sensual person yourself, your sensual child can drive you crazy.

Question from a mother:
What is the best response when your 20-month-old son takes your hand and places it on his penis (with or without an erection) and wants you to feel it?

It doesn't really matter whether you feel comfortable with a sensuous child or not – you can't change your nature. The important part in all of this is the child. He or she needs to be taught appropriate or socially acceptable behavior. Gently, kindly, remove the child's hands or pull yours away if the child has placed your hand on their private parts. Explain that this touching is not appropriate.

You might say, "Those are my private parts and I don't want people to touch me there." Or, "Joey, it is not appropriate to touch Auntie Sue's breasts, that is a private part. You can sit on Auntie's lap, but no fondling is allowed." Or, "It is not appropriate for me to touch your penis or kiss your private parts. Children and adults do not touch each other's private parts." You may have to repeat the message firmly, several times.

Of course, you will want to stay alert around this issue. Sometimes, a sudden interest in fondling and exploring is an indication of your child having been exploited or abused. Don't panic. Gently repeat the message about privacy and listen for any feedback. If the child responds in a positive way and discloses nothing, you probably have nothing to worry about.

These days, when we are all hypervigilant about abuse, our children need guidelines about appropriate behavior. No one wants their child to develop a reputation for being overly interested in other people's bodies and no one wants to put their child through an abuse investigation if it is not necessary.

A mother at one school told me about her five-year-old son asking where babies come from. The mother explained the whole process of intercourse and sperm meeting ovum. The little boy listened intently and then said, "Does the man have to have an invitation to do that?"

The Shy Child

Not all children are of the "sensuous" variety. Some children seem to be born with very shy natures or personalities. Parents sometimes suggest that it is because of birth order or gender, but who can really explain it?

We have all met children who are live wires at home with their family, but who are shy at school or at a party. Other children can be very quiet and seem to be extra sensitive at home, but active and engaging at school.

The children who worry me are the ones who seem to be very shy about sexual health. First, I am afraid that if the parent gives in to the child's hesitancy to be a part of a class, or if a parent excuses them from a presentation on sexual health, than that child is not receiving the education that will protect them. Will they come to a parent and ask a question? Will they be able to sort out which stories from the playground are true? Will they disclose an abusive situation? Will these children feel comfortable negotiating relationships as teens? Are they going to be assertive enough to make good decisions and will they be able to visit doctors as adults? I think parents are risking their children's lives when they shield them from sexual health teaching.

In the sidebars, I have included two stories that were written to me - one by a child who had no education, and one from a child who knew what to do because her mom had talked to her, made

One day I was walking home from school and a car pulled up and he asked me something and I went closer and I saw his penis and I havent ever told anybody → should I tell my parents?

her comfortable, and worked hard to help her daughter overcome her fears.

My good friend Heather Mains, a wonderful Montessori teacher, suggests that parents with shy children help them to be open and embrace difficult experiences as a wonderful challenge. If you can assure your child that he or she has your confidence that he can do it or she will be safer after, you give them a life-enhancing skill.

Ask yourself, "As a parent, when do I expect my child to get over being shy and super-sensitive? How and at what age will they do it?" It takes courage from the parent and the child to be joyfully engaged in the challenge, but surely, our children's lives are worth it.

Sexual Abuse

Not long ago, I ran into an old friend from my junior high days. I was telling her how much her father's wise words about life had meant to me. He had been my music teacher. She replied, "Yes, he was a good dad, too, but in his old age we really had to watch him." She went on to explain that his arteries had hardened when he was in his 80s and he had become chair bound. But although his legs had failed, his hands were everywhere. After several incidents of inappropriate fondling and groping of grandchildren, my friend and her siblings had to keep the children away from him.

This is not an uncommon story and it represents a situation which most families who are faced with it find difficult to handle. I know that caregivers rage about poor old folks who don't receive many family visits, but no one knows what went on in that family when the children were growing up, or what goes on now when grandchildren visit.

One time when I was at a store a man pulled me over the counter and kissed me, my mom got the police over and they went to see him

Of course, I am not suggesting that all grandparents become abusers, but awareness is the key and your child deserves your vigilance and protection.

Sometimes I hear stories about grandparents in a different context. Parents have told me that everyone knew that "Dad" had been an abuser when he was in his 30s and 40s. It may have been a family secret, or he was charged but acquitted, or he served time. But now he is in his old age, and surprise, surprise, he is still abusing! Unfortunately, jail time or advancing years do not always cure an offender. Grandpa could still be offending.

The "family secret" cases are the hardest to deal with because the conspiracy of silence keeps the whole family from learning about abuse. Sadly, it usually keeps the family from talking in a healthy way with the children. This puts the children in double jeopardy. Not only are they unprotected by ignorance around sexual health, but they are unprotected from grandpa. Even sadder is the fact that the wife, who couldn't or wouldn't protect her own children, is now also unable to protect her grandchildren. Some families have persuaded themselves that it is safe for grandpa to babysit because grandma is there.

Be aware, be vigilant, protect your children. They are the most important people in your life, not your parents or your in-laws. Your children come first.

There's Always a Reason

Remember that children never ask questions out of the clear blue. They have either heard something or something has happened – if not, they wouldn't be asking the question.

You might begin by gently asking where they heard about the word or activity.

Sometimes kids tease each other with words or names that none of them truly understand and, as casual and unconcerned as your child may seem to be, they can be concealing a great deal of pain or terror underneath a bland expression.

It is not unusual these days for young children to use words like virgin, sexy, humping, gay, lezy, (and worse), plus any number of slang words and expressions that are local to that school or neighborhood. Be honest if you don't know the word or don't have an answer to the question, and don't lie or evade or go on a tirade about them spending time with "undesirable" kids.

I think it is especially important in the primary years to remember that children sometimes ask mechanical-type questions because something has happened to them.

The following is a sad story, but it makes the point very well.

A mother phoned me in tears one autumn day. She had just discovered that her seven-year-old son had been abused that summer by a 12-year-old boy who lived in their neighborhood. When she asked her son why he had not told her at the time, he said, "I tried to tell you, Mom. Remember that day I asked you if guys put their wieners in other guys' bums? You said that only dirty men did that, and I didn't want you to think that I was dirty."

This mother discovered the abuse only because her son contracted a serious infection. As parents, we must not let homophobia put our kids in danger.

Of course, the next time your child asks a question, you must be careful not

How come some parents, when you tell them that some one (friend, relative) is sexually abusing you, they don't believe you?

to overreact. Having read the above story, your first instinct may be to grab your child by the shoulders and demand to know, "What has happened?" Stay calm, give some basic scientific information, watch their response, ask if they have further questions, and always remind yourself that if they are old enough to ask the question, they are old enough for the answer.

If they seem satisfied with your answer, compliment them on their question and leave the door open to revisit the topic. "If you want to know more sometime, be sure to ask me again. I'm really proud of you and your questions."

AIDS for Primaries

In my experience, the children who are most frightened about the illness called AIDS (acquired immune deficiency syndrome) are the preschoolers and the primaries. I think that is because they are exposed to the same news broadcasts, movies, and television programs as everyone else, but no one thinks to talk to them. Parents find it easier to talk with older children about such a frightening disease, and older children are articulate enough to ask questions. The very young don't always have the skills or the vocabulary to present their fears.

Some parents are terrified to provide information or to answer questions because of their own terror of AIDS. One mother asked, "How in the world do you ever begin to explain AIDS to an eight-year-old? My son keeps asking me because of news reports."

This mom thought that she'd have to explain homosexuality to her son; she was still thinking of AIDS as people did in 1980!

A mother told me about her third grade son, in tears after school, telling her that he was dying of AIDS.

When she asked him if he knew how people got AIDS he said, "Yes, I do. All the kids at school say you'll get AIDS if you don't wear a condom... And, Mom, I haven't been wearing a condom!"

Once I explained to her and to a room full of parents that what children really want to know is, "Am I in any danger?" she and the others visibly relaxed.

The most important information to give your children, and older ones, is that they are not in any danger. People acquire the HIV (human immunodeficiency virus) when they have sex with infected people, or when they use contaminated needles to inject drugs or share drugs. Reassure your child that since they are not having sexual intercourse or sharing needles, they have nothing to fear. Before scientists knew about HIV and the illness called AIDS, some people got the virus from blood transfusions. Now the blood is tested, so children shouldn't worry about acquiring the HIV in this way either.

Sometimes children hear that babies are born with HIV and can get sick with AIDS. It is important to reassure the young child who is concerned that they may have HIV or AIDS that only babies born to parents who are HIV infected are at risk. Since you (their parent) were not infected when the child was conceived, they don't have to worry.

There are some marvelous books that have been written to explain AIDS to preschoolers and older children. These can be very helpful, especially for those families who have a member who is living with an HIV infection. Two excellent books for preschoolers and primaries, both by Dr. Margaret Merrifield, are *Come Sit By Me* (Women's Press) and *Morning Light* (Stoddart).

Pre-puberty Information

Primary children need a few basic facts about puberty changes in advance of their own puberty for two reasons. First, they need to know a bit about what to expect so that if they are among the "early starters," they will not be frightened by the changes and can share and even celebrate them with their parents.

Second, there will be early starters in their peer groups at school, at summer camp, among their cousins, and so on. Children who do not know what more informed peers are talking about can feel isolated and even be ostracized by their peers.

So grab the teachable moments. It might be a good time to talk about toiletries, for example, while you're putting away the groceries you just purchased. "Sanitary pads, tampons: these go in the bathroom cupboard. By the way, do you know what they are for and how I use them?" Don't take, "Oh yeah, I know, Suzy told me," for an answer. Ask what Suzy said or what, *exactly*, does the child know? "The deodorant goes by the shower. Do you think you might need your own deodorant one of these days?" (See the next chapter for "the science of sweat.") Sometimes seven-year-olds need deodorant and eight-year-olds might be having nocturnal emissions and menstruation. There might be some breast budding (a little growth behind the nipple) as early as age seven, and sometimes pubic hair begins to sprout in second or third grade.

If you have any concern, please consult your doctor. There are some children who do have what is called precocious puberty and they need to be seen by specialist doctors and clinics.

I was teaching in a third grade classroom and encouraging girls to ask a the school office if they needed a sanitary pad.

"They will be very glad to help you," I said. "Everyone knows about periods."

"Even me?" asked one little boy in amazement.

The child beside him sighed and said, "Yes, even you, Bradley. You just learned about it now."

***

I was showing some primaries sanitary pads and one boy asked, "Is that a mini pad like on TV?" Before I could say yes, another child asked, "Do they make Mickey pads for boys?"

Bedtime Sharing

Here's a bit of practical advice about talking with primaries. Bedtime is often a great time to read a book together about some aspect of reproduction or how the human body works.

This is a good time to hear about worries from school, daycare, or a television show they saw or heard about. A back rub or foot massage almost always enhances sharing and the security that is needed to tell deep secrets and hidden fears. It also establishes the practice of sharing which can carry you both through later teenage years safely.

Caution

Some parents do not take this stage seriously enough. They do not appreciate that the child is growing up and is no longer a toddler. These parents need to appreciate the mechanical questions, the child's quest for "engineering" information, and the need to grow past the baby talk. Perhaps the following incident will illustrate this point.

In a third grade classroom, when I was talking about the penis delivering the sperm, the children all spoke at once, saying, "Oh, that's having sex," and giggling as usual. One boy, who was also giggling, spoke up and said, "My mom and I have sex all the time."

My knees went weak and the teacher's face drained of color.

The boy rushed on to say, "Yeah, we call it sexing when I sit on her lap and kiss her."

The teacher and I were both flooded with relief, and the other students laughed at him, but my point is this: that mother was very, *very* fortunate. The teacher told me later that the child's statement would have obliged her to call the child protection folks and to report the "disclosure" if he had not explained what he meant. It is not the teacher's job to ask for an explanation or to seek to question the child.

After school that day, the teacher telephoned the mother to tell her what had happened. The mother was embarrassed, but explained that she had thought it was "cute" behavior. She didn't want her boy "to know the facts of life and grow up too fast!" This lad was nine years old and no longer a baby.

I hear shame in that mom's behavior and great immaturity on her part. Her behavior was not fair to her son. Not only did she come very close to being the subject of a child abuse investigation, but she left the door open for her son to be teased by the other students and for stories to go home about her son to the other families.

Too many parents assume that because their children are innocent or uninformed, all other children that age are as well. In fact, your child may be the only one who doesn't have good information and a sensible approach in his or her group, from preschool onward.

A Final Word for "Engineers"

If a child's mechanical curiosity is not respected and nurtured, if it is squelched and he is ignored or she is ridiculed, it resurfaces throughout their lives.

Sometimes we feel very shy about admitting our curiosity and we repress it, endangering ourselves in the process. Let me tell you about one father who came to his son's fourth grade class and was quite hostile.

He told me he didn't believe sex education should be taught in elementary schools and he told me about some alarming rumors that had been spreading in the community about my presentations. I listened to his tirade, but had no time to reply since the students were waiting.

After the lesson, the children went for lunch and I asked the father how he felt now.

"I never had much more than three years at school," he began, "and if I had heard you when I was nine, my whole #@!!&* life would have been different!"

Before I could say a word, he rushed on. "So I've got a couple of questions for you. Why can't we still breathe out of our bellybuttons?" Then, in reference to my comments about nocturnal emissions, he asked, "If you never slept, would you fill up with sperm and explode?"

Blessing should rain down on this wonderful man forevermore. He asked his questions and he expected me to answer him with all the science that I had. It was one of my proudest moments.

As I tell the children, you never want to run out of questions or stop asking them. *And* there is no such thing as a dumb question – not in body science!

Primary
Checklist

Your primary child needs to know

- everything the preschoolers need to know, plus;
- the following scientific words: urine, stool, bladder, urethra (tube draining the bladder);
- the distinction between the digestive and reproductive systems;
- full information about menses and nocturnal emissions;
- basic/introductory information about body changes at puberty.

4

Intermediates
The "Gross-me-outers"
(Fourth Grade – Seventh Grade)

---

why do you have
to talk about sex
because it is so disgusting

how long does
puberty take?

What if I want to go to
bed early but I have
lots of homework to do?

Can women with
small breast give out milk
as women with big & the same
breast? amout of

I love the intermediate group most. They are so grossed-out they make me laugh, yet they are the most curious about sexual health and are very easy to teach once trust is built.

They write me anonymous notes: "Aren't you embarrassed to be such a pervert?" "Did you choose this job?" "Do you get paid to do this job?"

This is such a crucial age. It is our last chance to really teach them about sexual health.

The crucial work that they do at this stage to become sexually healthy adults is to develop their own personal boundaries and the modesty that our society expects around our sexuality.

This is usually the age when they begin to demand privacy, first for themselves, then for others. You may have a child who scandalized the neighborhood with his preschool quest for nudity at all times. Now, suddenly, he is not only in the bathroom combing his hair, but the door is locked, bolted, and barricaded. He may still come in, sit down, and talk to you while you sit on the throne, struggling with constipation, but no one is allowed in when *he* is in the bathroom.

Gradually, when intermediates are allowed to develop and maintain their own privacy, they begin to honor others' need for privacy too. Sexually mature people know their own boundaries and respect the boundaries of other people.

Sadly, this is also the age group that is most often sexually abused – with profound consequences. If children are not effectively treated after abuse, they tend to go in one

---

One mother told me about the shyness beginning in her nine-year-old son.

"Mom, the grossest thing, you know how the man puts his penis in the woman's vagina?"

"Yes, but it's really not gross," replied the mom.

"No, Mom, the grossest thing is...some guys like it!"

of two directions. The first is to build so many personal boundaries around themselves that they never have joyful, fully satisfying adult relationships; the second direction or inclination is to develop no boundaries at all, either for themselves or anyone else. An extreme example of this is that lack of boundaries among prostitutes and pornographers who come from abusive backgrounds.

Some adults have poor boundaries themselves and have no concept of respecting their children's boundaries.

Sometimes children tell me that they cannot bring friends home after school, "because my dad sits on the couch watching television in his underpants." When the child complains, the father (or mother) says, "It's my couch, my house, my television, and my privilege to wear whatever I like."

This is an adult who is immature; a mature adult would put the child's needs first and honor the child's quest for privacy. It is the *child's* home too and *they* need to experience respect for themselves at home before they can learn to respect the privacy of others.

Here's another example of poor boundaries. A third grade child turns up at school wearing a T-shirt that says, "Wine me, dine me, 69 me." Whoever bought the shirt and allowed her to wear it has poor boundaries. Not only is that adult disrespectful of society's boundaries, but they are violating the child's right to be safe. She is being set up for some hurtful questions and teasing at school, and she is also vulnerable to abuse or exploitation.

Many teens and adults who wear inappropriate clothing have not had an opportunity to develop the modesty and boundaries that are considered to be appropriate. Sadly, when they were younger, their parents were probably immature too. It all becomes an unhealthy cycle.

Children *need* parents and siblings who respect boundaries. One mom told me about a very puzzling conversation that she had with her nine-year-old daughter. The girl said she felt sorry that boys didn't have pajamas.

The mom replies, "Boys *do* have pajamas."

"Well, why doesn't Daddy?"

"Daddy has a lovely pair of pajamas hanging in the closet."

"Well, why doesn't he wear them?" the daughter asked in frustration.

These parents need to understand that their daughter is asking that her dad wear something when she meets him in the bathroom or hall. In my opinion, he should be able to sleep nude (he'll have healthy, cool testicles); the daughter is not likely hanging out in her parents' bedroom anymore. But he does need to wear the pajama bottoms outside the bedroom. If no one respects privacy at home, then children don't expect it outside their homes.

Although intermediate children can become quite shy, they may not remain as prudish as they are at nine or ten, once they become older. One dad said that when his daughter was ten years old, she demanded that everyone stop appearing naked in the "public" hallways between bedrooms and bathrooms. He and his wife began to wear robes, and continued to wear them until their daughter left for university.

A year later, home for the summer, the daughter appeared nude in the hall. Dad, in his robe, says, "Nice body, Julie."

"Thanks, Dad," she said, without any shyness at all.

Of course, if Granny is visiting, robes are appropriate. We all need to respect others' boundaries, especially when they, or we, are guests.

Unfortunately, as I've said, many adults are stuck at the intermediate stage because of abuse and lack of treatment. Others can feel stuck in the shy, embarrassed stage because they grew up in homes that may have been physically nurturing, but totally repressed around sexual health. It is terribly hard to grow beyond the maturity level of your parents, your school, and/or your society.

Explaining Pregnancy

Children aged nine to 12 are fascinated by pregnancy and have a million questions about how the baby grows inside the mother. They have even more questions about miscarriages, abnormalities, multiples, handicaps, and congenitally joined twins.

This immense curiosity is fueled by media sensationalism. The supermarket tabloids are a likely source of information for this age group. Intermediates don't have the knowledge or experience, however, to think clearly and to recognize the nonsense when it appears. Unfortunately, many parents also lack knowledge and will collude with the child's muddled information.

Here's a question I commonly receive: "Why do people have to take their clothes off?" The joking "scientific" answer is that the man cannot put his penis into the woman's vagina if they both have their pants on – or at least not easily. I think the bigger question here is embarrassment about nudity. Even adults who are stuck at this level refuse to undress fully during lovemaking. It is always worthwhile to impress upon intermediates that if they are too embarrassed to be naked or to undress in front of their partner, they are not ready for sex.

When you kiss with boys can we get pregnant

Other questions revolve around kissing, hugging, holding hands, toilet seats, bathtubs, and sleeping with someone as ways to get pregnant. This age group tries so hard to put things together for themselves, and while the attempt is admirable, without factual information it can be dangerous.

Explain that simply sleeping with someone will not cause pregnancy; sperm have to be placed in or very near the vagina.

"Making love" is another euphemism that is sometimes confused with hand-holding and hugging and kissing. Not everyone uses the term to refer to sexual intercourse.

The popular term "lost a baby" is another confusing expression for intermediates, on several levels. One girl asked her mother, after hearing family gossip, where Mrs. Jones had lost her baby. Her mom said she'd lost it at the hospital. Later, the girl asked, in tears, why Mrs. Jones hadn't gone back to find her baby, and begged her mom to "never stop looking for me if I get lost."

Many children hear about miscarriages via family gossip or ordinary news sharing among families and neighbors. The emergency-type hospital television shows are also incredibly graphic, but not always educational.

I like to help children understand, first, that they may not have received good information. Then I try to be honest with them.

Sometimes we know why a mother miscarried or had a handicapped baby. When I have asked children to brainstorm a list of potential harms to unborn babies, they have been remarkably accurate. They easily come out with alcohol, drugs, and smoking. Sometimes they know about poor nutrition, and they often talk about violence, accidents, and a mother being ill herself. I encourage them to avoid as many of these hazards as possible when they are growing up.

you can still have baby when you only sleep together instead of having sex.

It's important not to let children leave the discussion, however, thinking that all pregnancy misfortunes result from carelessness. Doctors and scientists don't know, always, why some anomalies occur and there are still many mysteries to be solved when it comes to conception, pregnancy, and birth.

Multiple births and congenitally joined or conjoined twins fascinate all of us, but most of all the media. Reports concerning the most babies, the largest, the smallest, the most pre-term baby all add to school-yard discussions.

Help your child to understand that fraternal twins come from two separate ova and two separate sperm. We don't know why the ovary sends out two or more ova at once, except that it is more likely to happen when the woman takes fertility drugs. Fraternal twins might be either boys, or girls, or one of each. They do not always look alike or grow alike.

Identical twins or multiples happen when *one* sperm fertilizes an ovum and, for some unknown reason, it splits into two or more babies. If the ovum does not separate completely, they are left joined together somewhere and they are called conjoined twins. Identical twins are always the same gender because there is only one sperm and that sperm carries the male or female chromosomes.

Is it because of sex sometimes the baby is deformed or dose it happing in your stomach from beer or wine?

How are identical twins produced?

Puberty

Intermediates are also going through puberty and have an enormous need for information about their changing bodies and emotions.

Parents say that they are more than willing to give information, but most do not start early enough. The best time to begin puberty information is whenever the questions come. Even preschoolers will ask, "Will I have bigger breasts when I grow up?" or "Will I have hair down there?" or "Will I need a tampon when I am bigger?" A simple "Yes" is a great way to start.

I remember a single father telling me about one day that started "horribly." He said he was nagging his four-year-old to eat her breakfast so that he could get her to preschool. She was engrossed in a Barbie doll and finally asked, "Dad, when I grow up, will I have boobs like these?"

The man told me that he just "freaked." "I mean, what next?" he said. "Why does a four-year-old need to know that? What was I supposed to say?"

If girls have small breasts now will they develope later.

"Yes, now eat your breakfast," seems to me like it would have been an appropriate answer. What I hear from this father is shame and an awful lot of emotional baggage that he's dragging around.

It is very helpful for pre-puberty children if their parents give information about puberty changes *before* they happen.

For instance, many boys develop small breasts during puberty. They need to know that this is normal and that, when their rib cage grows to adult size, those little breasts will spread out and not be so noticeable.

So many boys have told me that they were worried sick. "I'm turning into a girl," or "I've got breast cancer and I'm going to die." One 12-year-old boy was so relieved to hear me talk about this normal mammary development, he shouted out in front of all his classmates, "Yes! (Hand gestures, thumbs up.) This has been the best day of my entire life. I thought I was dying!"

His teacher and friends all laughed with him, but I wanted to cry. How long had he been walking around thinking he was dying? When I asked the whole class if they would ever share that fear with their parents, there was a unanimous, horrified "No" from these seventh grade students. Several said, "My parents don't talk to me about these changes, so I think I'm not allowed to talk to them." Others reflected our society's fear of cancer. "My mom would be sad if I got cancer and I don't want her to be sad, so I'll not tell her."

A family physician who attended one of my seminars for doctors told me that, just the day before, an 11-year-old boy had turned up in her office to ask her if he had breast cancer. He had not been able to voice his fears at home, so he'd made his way to the doctor, alone, to ask.

Do you have breast cancer if one brest grows bigger than the other?

Another student told me that she'd had an aunt die of breast cancer a few months before and was afraid to say anything about her own fears when she developed the hard node behind her nipple (which is normal for youngsters). She was afraid – terrified – that she'd have to have surgery and chemotherapy.

Sometimes your breasts hurt for no reason, why?

While you're at it, don't forget to explain that breasts can grow unevenly for a while, and that soreness is simply "growing pain." Of course, a visit to the doctor may reassure the child and can be helpful.

For girls, it is also helpful to point out that size doesn't matter. Adult women have breasts to feed babies and small breasts make just as much milk as large ones.

Hygiene at Puberty

For some strange reason, when children begin puberty, they perspire much more than they did before, but they also become allergic to soap and water!

Many have told me that their parents are constantly sniffing them and shouting, "You stink. Get into that shower!" Then, they tell me, they go into the bathroom, turn on the water, but they don't get under it. They sit on the toilet and read a comic.

One boy confessed that his mother had finally discovered that he wasn't showering because his hair wasn't wet. So now he stands outside the tub, gets a bit of water on the top of his head, and rubs it in. Then, in common with most of his peers, he sprays deodorant on and exits smiling.

My task is to explain the science of sweat to this group. Here's how I do it: "When perspiration comes out of your pores, it is clean. It doesn't smell. Within seconds, however, bacteria will appear from all over the neighborhood and will take up residence in your sweat. Bacteria smell! You must wash them off every day. If you put deodorant on top, you're gluing the bacteria from days before to yourself. More will come today and you will smell terrible."

After a wet dream, should someone wash up.

At this point, I often see kids smelling their armpits, or they will put their whole face inside their sweatshirts to smell themselves. This is what I tell them: "You may smell lovely to yourself, you're now used to the smell, but others are waving their hands in front of their noses and saying, 'Who smells around here?' You must wash your armpits every day. Some families cannot afford hot showers for everyone every day, but washing is essential. You can put deodorant on after washing if you like, but never put deodorant on top of stink you've already got – you'll smell ten times worse."

Don't forget to remind boys and girls about washing genitals too, and especially about rinsing away the smegma. It is heartbreaking when I am approached by a group of students (usually boys) who say, "Meg, there is this one person (almost always a girl) who really smells. Could you go and talk to her?" Sadly, it is a child or teen who has never had this science lesson and simply does not know.

Voice Changes

Voices change during puberty – girls' voices too. Sometimes it happens slowly over several months and sometimes it seems to happen overnight.

Body and Pubic Hair

Body hair grows in during puberty. Some children begin growing underarm hair and pubic hair in second grade, others not until late in high school.

It won't take children long to notice that women often shave their underarms and legs while males seem to take great delight in hairy armpits, chest, and leg hair.

If we are scientific, we know that shaving the armpits reduces underarm odor. We must respect people's personal preferences, however, and it is good to

How long can pubic hair get

***

A single mom said that her ten-year-old son had become very cranky and withdrawn. She thought it might be puberty.

That evening he called her into his bedroom, pulled down his shorts, and said, "Do you think this is enough pubic hair for a guy my age?"

"Yes," she stammered.

Obviously relieved, the son said, "Whew! I was so worried," and hopped into bed, all crankiness gone.

point out to children that it is a personal choice whether to shave any body hair.

That being said, if your daughter wants to shave her armpits and/or her legs, put aside the old-fashioned idea that shaving causes the hair to grow in darker, coarser, and more abundantly. It simply isn't true. It really doesn't matter, and rather than allow this to become a power struggle, buy her an electric razor and let her get on with it. Put succinctly, "Don't sweat the small stuff." Believe me, there will be far more important struggles to come. Give her some pride and ownership in her developing body, and celebrate the invention of the electric razor!

There is tremendous anxiety among pubescent children about pubic hair. The uneducated all seem to believe that it will be black for every single person, curly from the first hair, and grow in on their 21st birthday. I believe that this anxiety is the fault of the large department stores that send out full-color catalogs and flyers to advertise their underwear. None of the models have pubic hair sticking out of the underwear. No wonder children worry about themselves! There are so many false images of the human body in advertisements.

Another mom told me about her nine-year-old daughter sobbing in the bath when she found her first pubic hair: "I'm too young to be a grown-up lady," she wailed. Mom reassured her that she had years of childhood left. Later, when the daughter emerged from the bathroom, her mom asked her if everything was okay.

"Oh yes, it's fine, Mom. I shaved it off!"

Pubescent children love to "play" with any information I provide about pubic hair and it is fun for adults to enjoy their playful questions as they erase their anxiety.

"Why does it grow between your legs?" "If you dye your head hair green, will your pubic hair turn green?" "If I shave my hair on my head in a Mohawk, will my pubic hair grow that way?" "My dad is going bald on top, is he going bald down there too?" and on and on. A common, sadder question I get is this: "I've been so worried about my pubic hair and I've pulled it out or shaved it off. Will it grow back?"

Testicular and Penis Growth

It takes boys about three years after the onset of puberty to grow their testicles to adult size. Many parents have said, "You know, I thought he might be going into puberty – the crotch of his pants has been filling out."

But the science that boys are often missing is that it takes eight to ten years after the onset of puberty to grow their penises to adult size. As a result, I get these strangled little voices saying, "I think my penis is shrinking." One of the most common anonymous questions I get from ten-year-old boys is, "What is the world's longest penis?" What they are really asking is, "What's the world's *smallest* penis, because I think I've got it."

Now, you probably didn't have to buy this book to learn what I'm going to say next, but I'll say it anyway. Preoccupation with penis size lasts a lifetime! The single most common complaint among healthy, middle-aged men is, "My penis is shrinking." Here's the good news. Your penis *does not* shrink in middle age; it's just that you grow a potbelly and you can't see as much of it anymore.

Here's some more penis science. Because boys (and girls) are often exposed to pornography, and therefore see the "stars" with giant penises, it is good to ask them to think like scientists: No one has a giant penis in real life. The penis fills up with blood to get erect. If you had one longer than the norm and it filled up with blood, you'd faint and it wouldn't do you any good. If there really were men with giant penises, they'd be holding up lampposts all over town.

The penises that children and adults see in pornography are "add-ons" that can get erect and shoot sperm five miles – but they are not real. Or, like some breasts, they have been surgically augmented and, when you think about it like a scientist, those augmented ones are not "real" either.

I think it is a sign of our society's great immaturity that some people feel that they must have that kind of surgery. It can make a great discussion topic with your children and teens. This could also be a superb time to talk about the abundance of false images of the human body, and about the manipulation of what is beautiful, handsome, and attractive. Grab that teachable moment with joy, respect for your child's ideas, and don't forget to laugh with them too.

Just to add to everyone's scientific knowledge here, flaccid or soft penises can be all different sizes – long, short, fat, thin, even curved. As long as they work without any discomfort, they're fine. When penises get erect, they are all about the same size (between five and a half, and seven inches long; that's 14–18 cm if you're using metric).

Remember that the penis is designed to deliver sperm and that you only need about two inches to do that. Anything you get after that is decoration.

On a more serious note, if you have any questions about your son's penis size, do ask your doctor. It is very rare, but occasionally, a boy will have a micropenis, a condition for which there is treatment available.

Testicular Health

I am often met by blank stares when I talk about testicular health, and yet testicular cancer is now one of the leading causes of death in young teens and adults. Let me say loudly and clearly that our young men don't need to die! Testicular cancer can be easily treated if it is found in its early stages.

Young teens and adults need to know how precious their testicles are and that it's a good idea to examine them on a regular basis. An excellent time for your teen (and every other adult male in the family) to examine his testicles is when he takes a shower. The testicles should feel smooth, like a peeled, hard-boiled egg. If he finds any bumps, or anything that feels like a grain of salt, have a doctor examine him

You said that all men have about the same size penis, then what are the ones in movies, cause they all look so long?

just to be sure. Don't worry about bumps or irregularities in the skin of the scrotal sac itself. Remember to point out that one testicle is usually smaller than the other and that when he stands one hangs lower in the sac. If nature had placed them exactly side by side, they'd knock together when he walked! Be prepared for gales of laughter and please join in. But do, also, stress the seriousness of testicular health and safety.

Phone your nearest cancer agency or public health unit and ask them to send you a half dozen pamphlets on testicle examinations and how to do them. They are free, so you can hand them out to other testicle owners and save lives.

Another Word or Two about Menstruation

I don't believe that there is much need to belabor the intricacies of menstruation with young girls. I concentrate on the health of the process. The lining or endometrium is shed each month; I try not to use phrases such as "cleaning itself" because I think such phrases suggest that it is dirty. As long as the female has no infections, the flow is clean. Of course, the girl must wash her vulva daily, or bacteria can cause the flow on the outside to have an odor.

How big is the average penis

What happens if you get cancer in your testicles?

WHY DOES ONE TESTCAL HANG LOWER THAN THE OTHER?

IF YOUR BALLS ARE DIFFERENT SIZES WHAT DOES THAT MEAN? (NOT SAYING I HAVE THAT)

The unfertilized ovum does not come out with the flow. It begins to dissolve 12 hours after it comes out of the ovary. It is pure protein and her body simply reabsorbs the protein, usually from the abdominal cavity. The ovum may never enter the fallopian tubes. Another common misunderstanding, usually from the very old-fashioned films we saw when we were at school, in which the uterus filled the screen, is that menstruation is connected to ovulation, and ovulation to menses. Most females miss ovulating two or more months a year. They still have their periods, but that is not proof that they have ovulated. And sometimes females are ovulating, but not menstruating.

When a girl begins to menstruate, she can be very irregular. It usually takes two to four years to become regular and some women never become regular. For the most part, whatever your body does is healthy for you.

Can you have 1 or 2 periods and then stop?

Do you get cramps when you have a period?

Cramps and painful periods may be caused by low calcium and magnesium levels. Many girls cut back on dairy products because of the calories and then become very low in calcium. I encourage the use of natural remedies before pharmaceutical aids. Try a calcium/magnesium tablet or two with a cup of hot milk chocolate, tea, or coffee with lots of milk. The heat, calcium, magnesium, and caffeine will all help, often promoting urination, which helps too. She may need to be on regular calcium and other supplements, including vitamin B12, especially if she's experimenting with the type of vegetarianism that does not include eggs or dairy products.

Girls (and boys) as young as six have been found to be obsessing about their bodies and secretly dieting or refusing to eat. Please make certain that your own preoccupation with your body, diets, and binges, don't set an example for your child. You can also protect your child from uneducated relatives' remarks to your child about weight gain, puppy fat, pinching an inch, and so on. I advise children that it is natural to "plump up" just before a growth spurt. I advise adolescents who *do* have a potbelly or spare tire to tell whoever is doing the commenting that they need a science lesson.

Menstrual health is too often compromised in girls by lack of adequate nutrition, lack of exercise, constipation, and the unrealistic body images found in girls' magazines.

Fathers can be especially supportive in the preteen and teen years by demonstrating healthy eating patterns themselves, by promoting fresh air and exercise for both sons and daughters, and by continuing to be psychologically supportive of the prepubescent or pubescent child. Too many dads withdraw their affection and attention, especially from daughters, as puberty approaches.

One woman told me about her dad, who, years ago and in his own peculiar way, *didn't* abandon her. Left alone, and raising four teenage boys and herself at age 12, he said to her out of the blue one day, "Have you started yet?"

"Yes," she responded shyly, eyes down.

"All right, I know how to take care of that."

He drove away in the car, returned an hour later carrying in boxes and boxes of sanitary pads, and stuffed them under her bed. "There," he said. "Now you have lots of supplies and your brothers don't need to know."

In a fifth grade class laughing about how ridiculous the pad ads are on TV:
Girl: Oh yeah, I saw them, but I didn't know what they were for. When I got my first period I was so scared. I said to my mom, "I have blood down there and I have a terrible headache." Mom handed me a pad and said to put it on in the bathroom – I put it on my forehead because it was way more painful than my vagina.

Years later, in fun, she reminded her dad of his trip to the store and said, "Dad, I've just run out of supplies, could you get me some more?"

Girls need their dads! Don't abandon her.

Another Word about Nocturnal Emissions

I obviously did not give enough information to one third grade class about boys' wet dreams. One eager little fellow put up his hand and said, "Well, my brother is 13 and he doesn't have those wet dreams yet."

I said, "You know, they are kind of private and perhaps he has had them, but he hasn't told you."

"Nope," he said with true conviction. "I sleep in the bottom bunk and nothing has poured down on me yet."

Do people get wet Day Dreams.

Only one spoonful of milky white liquid comes out. It doesn't flood the bed. Most boys say it feels like extra sweat. They need to know that the semen is clean and that nocturnal emissions are healthy. It is their body practicing for being grown-up.

By the way, sometimes boys feel very guilty about nocturnal emissions because they think it implies they've had a sexy dream. He doesn't have to be dreaming, just deeply asleep. Sexy dreams are normal, too, but they don't have to be associated with nocturnal emissions.

Wedgies and Purple Nurples

What's a purple nurple?

In my travels around the country, visiting schools in urban and rural areas, I've become aware of two "tortures" that elementary and secondary students inflict on each other.

"Purple nurples," from pinching and twisting breast tissue and nipples, are very common, as are "wedgies," from pulling the pants up between the legs or even from hanging the child up on hooks by the belt. Both of these activities are technically sexual assaults – one person is interfering with another person's private parts – and are therefore also, technically, against the law.

I encourage children to yell loudly and to tell on the perpetrator if they are attacked in either manner. I encourage adults to protect children and to put an end to these practices.

When doctors first began to suggest that I educate kids about wedgies – because they can severely damage testicles – I had no idea that girls were attacked in this manner as well. But from the very first mention, girls began to "tell."

The genital area in both males and females is easily damaged. So is breast tissue. We all need to learn to keep our hands (and our feet) to ourselves. No interference with another person's body or clothing is allowed!

Body Image – It's about Being Accepted

Children are sensitive to the popular commercialized messages about the "ideal" body shape and size. Many children, even slender ones, worry, "Am I too fat?" Our children would feel more confident and have a better "sense of self" if they were certain they were loved for who they are, not for what they look like. There are good resources available that deal with food preoccupation, body image, and eating disorders. If you have a concern, see a doctor.

Emotional Development

Children have a unique opportunity to learn how to control their emotions during puberty, but they need adult assistance. Unfortunately, there are many adults who grew through puberty and lacked adult assistance themselves.

We need to welcome this time of emotional intensity and help them learn ways to cope. I tell kids, "It may be normal to have hormone attacks and to feel as if you are out of control, but it is not acceptable to punch holes in walls or to try to kill your brother. It is not his fault that you are in puberty and he deserves to live another day."

Most families report that supper is frequently a troublesome time. One child begins to fool around, there's lots of giggling, but then someone gets hurt and begins to cry. Then one of the participants gets angry and wants to kill!

I tell children that it is normal to get the "sads, glads, and mads" during puberty.

The glads are when you get the giggles and you can't stop laughing. They are contagious, too. One person gets a hormonal glad and their hormones call to everyone else. Soon the whole class is laughing and no one knows the cause.

The sads are when you become hypersensitive, every little thing bothers or worries you, you cry and don't know why. It feels as if you are alone, no one likes you, you're ugly, and so are your parents.

It always seems important to me to alert parents to this aspect of the sads. Don't take it personally, and despite what your child may say, this dislike of parents has nothing to do with your ethnic background, or your job, your interests, or your talents. *All* parents face weeks of sometimes intense dislike from their children. It is hormones, and if the truth be known, there are times when we parents don't like our children much either. Stay calm, rise above it, and take a moment to remember your own rebellious thoughts at that age.

There is a fine line between what might be called normal pubertal hormonally induced depressions, and depression that needs serious attention. Don't hesitate to seek help if you or your child is concerned. It may be that all you and your child need is a little bit of professional help to develop coping skills when the world seems pretty bleak and inhospitable. I do not believe in leaving kids to sort out their own problems for weeks at a time. I think that is abandoning children. If they can't sort it out in a few days, step in and offer help yourself, or seek help. That's what parents are for.

The mads are mostly about "homicidal" feelings and actions toward a sibling. Children often erupt in hoots and hollers of agreement when I raise this hormonal moment. They are so relieved that someone is talking about it. They tell me that they are often frightened of the intense feelings, physical strength, and the backlash of their parents. Simply put, "I know my family hates me and I hate myself when I explode. Why do I do it?" They feel ashamed and want to apologize, but don't know how to do it.

I talk to them about those feelings and get them to brainstorm ideas that will help them cope without killing their sibling and getting themselves deeper into trouble. In a classroom there are always children who stand out during these discussions, children who obviously have parents who have taught them well. Barbaric behavior is simply not tolerated by these parents, no violence is allowed, and neither is verbal abuse. There is liberal use of the "time out." It's all right to say, "Go to your room." Expect your child to welcome time alone: "This is not punishment, this is growing time. Listen to music, read, or write in a journal (here parents must promise not to snoop), write a letter to whoever has upset

My friend says that you are also very grumpy when you go through puberty is that true ???

Is a sadness spell when you think every thing seems to be going wrong?

what do you do if you feel guilty after you get mad but don't want to show it?

you or been unfair." Parents must be prepared to arbitrate with justice. Sometimes one child has a legitimate complaint about their sibling or their parent.

Parents may want to write to the child and point out how hard it is to arbitrate and be fair but firm. Sometimes parents need to apologize too, and writing it down can be tremendously helpful for both parent and child.

Physical exercise is a good outlet. Suggest that your child go for a run with your dog, shoot some baskets, hit some tennis balls, play hockey. I like to suggest to students that Wayne Gretzky probably had lots of mad attacks and shot pucks instead of fighting at home. "Look where his hockey skills got him. You could use your mads to improve your talents and become rich and famous too!"

A Word about Bullying

But let me reiterate: too often, children suffer grave injustices at home, at school, and in their communities. We need to listen to them and help them to identify and to articulate their problems. Then we need to be there for them seeking justice. They are young. Don't abandon them.

Thank goodness our communities are now responding seriously to violence, bullying, and other intolerant behaviors. Children's self-esteem and sense of trust in the world can be badly damaged by the inappropriate actions of others, or by bystanders doing nothing to help the victim. When those things happen, the affected child is more likely to be vulnerable and to take more risks involving sexual health.

I would urge parents to support their children, as well as school and community programs that promote problem solving and zero tolerance for bullying.

If your child is the bully, find out why this is happening and use every resource available to get help for him or her.

Sleep and Sleep Disturbances

Having said that, let me suggest one more remedy for suppertime blues.

I like to tell children that scientists say that growth hormones are released in our bodies when we are deeply asleep. Therefore, all elementary students, especially, need extra sleep. In fact, probably each one is going to have a "heavy-duty-growing-night" at least once a week. I tell them that when parents are making supper, "They can take one look at you and tell if tonight is a heavy-duty-growing-night."

How do you think parents can tell? There is usually one child who says, "I don't know, but my dad takes one look, points his finger at me, and says, 'You are going to bed early tonight.'" One girl said recently, "Yeah, you know, your parents aren't really mad, they're really just trying to help you grow properly."

"Vegging out," watching television, not doing chores or homework, whining, crying, moaning, complaining about the supper, and most of all, trying to kill a sibling, are all signs of heavy-duty-growing-nights.

Adults sometimes get the sads, glads, and mads too, often in direct relation to the number the children have had lately.

If you are a very modern adult, you may have delayed your childbearing into your 30s or 40s. You may be in a second relationship with "his," "her," and "our" children, and by the time that you get all these children into puberty, you may be going through hormonal changes yourself. Some evenings we can get the whole family swinging from the chandeliers. Everyone needs to go to bed early! Sleep deprivation may be the biggest health hazard for everyone in the 21st century.

How long should you sleep a day?

I want to be serious, though. Some puberty age children can be plagued by sleep disturbances and be wide awake for hours after their normal bedtime.

Some children, especially those who are going through an active growth spurt, have night terrors. These usually happen as they are trying to sleep and they are overcome with irrational fears. They can cry, shake, cling, feel nauseated and plain terrified.

"What if there is an earthquake, a tidal wave, or some other natural disaster?" "What if you die, Mom or Dad, what would I do?" "What if I die?" "What if my dog dies, or what if I got a dog and then it died?"

News stories and television movies often trigger these fears, or some member of the child's extended family or community suffers a tragedy and sets them worrying.

My advice would be, first, to always treat the fear seriously. Exactly what could they do in an emergency? You may need to put an earthquake kit, or three, in place at your house. Plan with your child about who to call. Make a list of emergency numbers and include any relatives or friends that you would trust with your children. Walk them through an escape plan if there was a fire or a flood. Children can be enormously relieved to be given some power and autonomy in an emergency. Assure them that you trust them and are confident that they can cope.

Of course, it would be good to point out how minimal the risk of some disasters is. The West Coast might suffer an earthquake, but rarely a hurricane. Kansas and Saskatchewan will never have tidal waves to worry about, and so on. This can be most reassuring for the child.

When it comes to normal sleep patterns, parents need to recognize that all children do not have to have the same amount of sleep, just like adults. I do believe that children need a regular bedtime and that they should be in their beds, or at least in their bedrooms, at the same time every night, with reasonable exceptions for special occasions, of course.

But I also think that it could be unhealthy for them to be forced to lie in the dark for hours on end, unable to sleep. Perhaps they could have a bedside light on and be allowed to read for a bit, or do some writing or a craft in bed, or have the radio on.

In listening to parents for many years, I have come to believe that the parent whose own sleep patterns are radically different from their child's has the hardest time. I think that it is best to relax and allow children to discover, through puberty, their own best sleep patterns.

That does not mean that you should allow "night owl" children to be up, roaming the house and disturbing you. If you need ten hours of sleep, you need to tell them that, offer sleep inducers – calcium-rich bedtime snacks, grilled cheese sandwiches, hot milk drinks or warm baths, hot water bottles, a back or foot rub, a bedtime story – but then insist that they stay in their beds. Above all, they must be safe while mom or dad is asleep.

Marital Problems

One more worry that is common, and that often causes major sleep disturbances is, "What if you and Dad (or Mom) get divorced?" Remember that the paramount question in children's minds is, "What will happen to me?" Naturally, if you can, you will want to reassure them that a divorce is not on the agenda – *if you can*. Please don't lie to them if it is. If there is tension in your marriage, a lot of verbal or physical abuse, put yourself in the child's place; wouldn't you be frightened, scared to death, unable to sleep?

Reassure the child that none of your difficulties are his or her fault. Be honest about how hard it is sometimes. Seek professional help and don't settle for a relationship that gives your children night terrors and nightmares. Show them that mature adults can work it out.

You may need to seek counseling, and if your partner won't go, go alone. Be aware that there are some therapists who are very skilled and others who are not. Be a knowledgeable consumer. Don't continue with someone who is not helping. Just because your friend or clergyperson recommended the therapist doesn't mean that they will be good for you.

Some therapists only see couples together and some want the whole family involved. Either style is fine if it works. But the bottom line is the children and their right to grow and flourish in a healthy home. You chose to be a parent, or parents, and for at least 19 years, your children come first.

Putting children first can sometimes mean that a separation or divorce is necessary. There are toxic relationships that harm children, those that involve abuse of alcohol, drugs, or control (especially by violent means). Too many parents say, "It's okay, I am the one being battered, not my kids." But the sight of a parent being battered is terrifying for children. Leave, if it means a healthier life for your children and you.

When asked, sometimes children want their parents to separate, and they are willing to accept a lower standard of living, or a single parent situation, in order to have some peace and security and consistency in their lives.

Children and teens come first. That doesn't mean that they rule the roost or have complete control, but it does mean that adults who chose to be parents at *conception*, need to be brave, mature, and to provide a healthy, nurturing home.

Talk to your children, model maturity for them. It is a gift that you give your children that may save their lives one day.

STDs and Condoms for Intermediates

Most intermediates have heard about some of the sexually transmissible diseases, but they have many questions and a lot of misinformation.

Questions about hemorrhoids are very common from children when we talk about STDs. Perhaps it is the strange ads on television that have one woman saying to another, "When I had my last baby, I had hemorrhoids." Who knows, but many children and teens think that you get "swollen hemorrhoidal tissue" when you have sex!

Here's what I tell kids: "Let's think about this like a scientist. Hemorrhoids are varicose veins of the anus and they are aggravated by constipation. They have nothing to do with sex."

"Whew, what a relief," the children say.

Intermediates, like primaries, need reassurance that many STDs are only transmitted through sexual contact: "So if you are not sexually active, you have nothing to worry about."

I would suggest that parents be prepared to talk about STDs and to answer any questions that very curious and articulate intermediates have. They don't always understand documentaries or news reports on television.

Movies give confusing information, as do the afternoon talk shows. If the parent doesn't know about the show or the latest research that was on the news, it is hard to debrief it with the child.

Be aware, too, that the community's discussion about condom machines being in high schools has left many preteens convinced that the dispensing machines are already in every single secondary school. Furthermore, intermediates often believe that that means that every teenager is having sex and that as long as you use condoms, everything will be fine or guaranteed.

what causes Hemeroids

Children see wilder condoms on sale in novelty shops all the time and are full of questions about flavored condoms, glow-in-the-dark condoms, musical condoms, and full-body condoms. They report street entertainers who blow up condoms and, of course, they read the ads and gossip about condom shops.

why do the people sell condoms in washroom vending machines? / why are there glow in the dork condons?

It is fun to share the jokes with kids, but be sure to repeat this injunction: "No matter how colorful or intriguing the pictures are on discarded condoms, don't touch them when you find them outside."

You might want to make certain that your child or teen understands that condoms do not always work and that just because there might be dispensers in some schools, hotels, washrooms, and even in some cigarette machines, it does not mean that it is safe for teens to have sex. More importantly, it doesn't mean that all teens are sexually active. Most teens in Canada who are still attending school are not having sex and the numbers who are not having sex are increasing in the U.S. too.

If your preteen is asking for more information on STDs, please see the adolescent section (pages 118–119) and Chapter 10 on STDs (page 177). Some intermediates are ready for a lot of scientific information long before their peers.

Practical Tips

Rarely do adults deny the intermediate's need for support and acceptance, but we often fall short of providing these things in abundance because of our own immaturity. A good example is the parent who says, "Well, I tried to talk to him, or to give her a book, but they were so embarrassed that I got embarrassed and just left it."

If you've tried talking in the kitchen and they've said, "This is so gross, I'm out of here," remember that the best place to talk to 10- to 20-year-olds is in the car where they're a captive audience. Sure they may stuff their fingers in their ears, call you sick, stare silently out the side window for three straight hours, but keep on talking. They will never forget that car ride. Neither will you. Just remember, they're worth it.

In Vancouver, I often joke with my parent audiences and suggest that all families should drive to Seattle or Whistler at least once a year, the kids in the back seat (they don't have to look you in the face), and of course, after dark is even better.

Some fathers have told me that they have had good discussions in a boat while fishing. Unless the children can walk on water, they are captive! Others tell about campfire or tenting discussions, even discussions held while cleaning out the garage (it keeps the hands busy and eye contact at a minimum)! Never miss a teachable moment. Talk the talk and keep it going.

Intermediate
Checklist

Your intermediate child needs to know

- everything the previous age groups have learned, plus;
- all about body changes at puberty;
- basic information about STDs (see pages 177-187 for more information).

You should also discuss the following topics

- the false and exaggerated sexuality portrayed in pornography and the exploitation of participants (see page 159);
- the understanding that one doesn't *have* to be a sexually active teen;
- the distorted, popular, commercialized views of the "perfect body."

5

Adolescents
The People Who Don't Know
That They Don't Know
(Seventh Grade – Twelfth Grade)

If during sexual intercourse the penis is pulled out before ejacualation can the female get pregnant?

WHAT IS AN ORGAZIM?

Everyone saise to use a condom for safe sex but what if you want to have a baby?

Why would women take Viagra?

Teens face two big obstacles on their journey to becomingsexually mature adults – especially if they have not been educated about sexual health by their parents or schools before they reach their teen years.

First, they think that they are supposed to know all about sexuality by virtue of being 14. Movies, magazines, and television all promote the image of teens as boiling sexual machines. When they realize that they don't know something, they think it is not cool to ask questions. They worry that their friends will see that they don't know, and it may seem too cooperative to ask and actually participate in a discussion with parents. Detached silence is a form of rebellion common to adolescents who fear disclosure of ignorance.

It's not surprising, then, that in all my years working with teens, I have not met a single one who was enjoying an active sex life – not one! Like all of us, teens want to be loved and cared about. Most who are sexually active want someone's arms around them, someone to listen to them, someone to do things with them. But they don't want intercourse.

The boys' bodies are not ready; they ejaculate much too fast and then want to die of embarrassment. The girls rarely, if ever, have an orgasm. I always get questions from teenage girls about orgasms. They've never had one and are constantly asking, "Is that all there is – a wet spot and nothing more?"

> My boyfriend and I are having trouble having sex. I can't get an orgasm. The only thing that works is oral sex... Is there a trick to the orgasm thing.... It frustrates me sooo much.

There are two good books available called *The First Time*, Volumes 1 and 2 (Orca Books, 1995). They are in paperback and are inexpensive. They contain true stories of "the first time" that various well-known authors had sex, or tried to have sex. I recommend them for cautionary awareness among all teens!

The second problem teens face is that, because our society is sexually immature, no one talks openly about sexual health problems and teens are hampered by lack of experience. They often say, "I don't accept that problem or issue you are warning us about. I don't know anyone who is HIV positive, or who has had genital warts, or an unplanned pregnancy, so those problems do not exist, or they don't exist in my group or town or university..."

I like to ask them if they would tell anyone if they were going to a doctor for genital warts treatment. They slide down in their seats, put their hands over their faces, and say, "Oh no, I'd never tell anyone," – not even the partner who gave them the warts. Then I say to them, "Now do you see why you don't know anyone who has these problems?"

There are many adults who are stuck at the adolescent level; they believe that they know everything, or should know because they are over 19, or because they have had sex or babies and therefore should know it all. They don't ask questions, they don't read newspapers or magazine articles, they don't seek information. They don't know that they don't know.

Smoking

More and more we are coming to understand the sexual health problems caused by smoking. I tell boys that if they begin to smoke as young teens, and keep on smoking as adults, they'll damage their penises. They reply with a challenge: "Oh yeah? I know lots of guys who smoke and they don't have damaged penises."

"How would you know?" I ask. "Men don't come up to each other at the local donut shop and say, "Hey, buddy, I can't get it up anymore.""

Doctors say that most men with impotency problems don't even tell their physicians let alone anyone else.

Prior to 2000, boys would sometimes say, "Hey, Meg, put that on the cigarette packages: 'Smoking kills your penis.'" I always believed that we could wipe out smoking in short order if we had the sexual maturity to do that! Then, in 2000, Canadian cigarette packages began carrying the warning, "Tobacco use can make you impotent." Canada now has the lowest rate of smoking in the world.

Of course, smoking affects almost the entire body because of the many toxins in the cigarette. But it is the carbon monoxide (CO) that damages the penis especially. Carbon monoxide causes blood vessels to constrict and since the most vascular organ is the penis, it is seriously damaged when the blood can no longer flow into it to create an erection.

Studies have also shown alarming damage to sperm, related to greater incidence of miscarriage and children born with disabilities.

I find that boys are much more responsive to this information than we adults might expect. Most of them are truly interested in being good fathers and, naturally enough, in their own sexual health.

Unfortunately, the information about the serious and critical damage that nicotine does to girls' ovaries and fertility falls on deaf ears among girls who already smoke. They reply that they don't plan on having children and that they're going to continue smoking "because it keeps me thin." (The magazine ads all have slim, elegant looking women with cigarettes between their fingers – never in their mouths, because it doesn't look elegant there! And there is no smoke coming off the end of the cigarette or hanging in the air, of course, not since secondhand smoke has been implicated in health problems.) Teenage girls are the fastest growing group of smokers and they ignore or deny the attendant problems.

For instance, studies have shown that damage can be passed on to the second generation of female smokers. The woman with a grandmother who smoked, even when her own mother and she herself did not smoke, is 27 percent more likely to miscarry than a woman with no family history of smoking at all.

Girls do not always understand that they are born with their tiny egg cells, their ova, already established in their ovaries, unlike males who create new sperm every minute. Studies have also found that females who smoke have more uncomfortable pregnancies and more painful backaches and headaches, as well as more infections and vomiting.

Parents tend to think of the teen years as the time when children are most likely to begin smoking, not realizing that seven- and eight-year-olds are often encouraged to begin smoking, usually by slightly older cousins, neighbors, and brothers and sisters of friends.

Talk to your child about the perils of smoking. One mother did and she was very surprised by her 12-year-old daughter's response: "Some of my friends smoke and they usually offer me one, but I never take one. I tell them that my mom would kill me."

This mother, at first, was shocked at being portrayed as such an ogre. She quickly regained her perspective, however, and replied, "I'm very proud of you for saying that. I hope that you will also say that I am a bloodhound, I'll smell the smoke on you, in your hair and clothes, and I will track down the person who gave you the cigarette too."

Think about it. Cigarettes are illegal in most jurisdictions for kids – so is alcohol. If we saw 12-year-olds on the street drinking beer and getting drunk, we'd want to know who gave them the alcohol and we'd charge them. Why do we not react the same way at the sight of young people smoking? Some schools even designate a smoking area. Isn't this lunacy?

Many studies have shown that if a person doesn't smoke before they are 20, they are very unlikely to begin as adults. It is time to get serious about smoking, time to save our future generations. It is your grandchildren that you are saving when you insist on non-smoking children.

Setting Limits

Another task – often neglected – for parents of teens is that of setting limits, guidelines, or even firm ground rules. As I have said before, much of what we teach our children (and ourselves) about sexual health is really just good manners. Keep that in mind when you discuss curfews, guidelines, and bottom lines of behavior with your children.

Children and teens often tell me that they are secretly glad that their parents have firm rules and guidelines, or that they wish their parents had more of them. Some stories may suffice to illustrate this point.

One mother said that her 13-year-old daughter came home from school with a very short leather skirt that her friend had loaned her, "so I can show you and you can buy one for me." The mom took one look at it and said, "No, I will not buy you one, and you're not allowed to borrow it and wear it."

Tears followed. Then yelling, door slamming, and accusations: "You're so old-fashioned, you never let me do anything; everyone else is getting one," even, "I hate you." Eventually, she was sent from the table without supper. During the evening, she continued to reappear from her bedroom, begging, cajoling, and crying. Finally she was ordered to bed and told to go to sleep.

In the morning, she stomped off to school, skirt in the bag, still saying that her mom was the worst mom in the world.

But what a change at four that afternoon. "Mom, I'm sorry about last night. I didn't really want the skirt, but I had to go to school and tell Sherrie that I had had tantrums and screamed at you all night and you still wouldn't let me have the skirt."

Don't be afraid to hold your ground. You may not get thanks as quickly as this mother did, but they *will* be thankful.

Alcohol and drugs are closely connected to teens' sexual activity. So talk with your youngsters frequently about that. "If I let you go to this party, what will you do if there is alcohol there, or if drugs are produced?" Go through your worst-case scenario; tell them about your worst fears. Ask them, "If you were a parent, what would you want your kid to do?"

Here's another story. One father told me that when his son received his first invitation to a mixed party, he (the father) was very careful. He phoned the classmate's mother to ask for details. "Yes, I will be there at all times. Yes, I am aware of young teens. I am a child psychologist; there is nothing to worry about."

The father drove his son to the party and reminded him (despite the host mother's assurances) that he was to phone if there were any problems. "I will come and get you and I will not be mad."

Two hours later, the son was on the phone. "Dad, I'm at a mall pay phone, please come and get me. The party was awful."

The father arrived, trying to quell his own panic. As the boy hopped into the car, the dad asked, "What happened?"

His son said, "It was awful. Everyone was drunk, some kids were throwing up and being really weird. I sneaked out of the house and walked until I found a pay phone."

The father was shaken. "But where was Dr. Jones? She promised me she'd be there. Where did the alcohol come from?"

"Oh, Dr. Jones gave everyone wine or beer. She said that she knows that kids need to experiment and she said that it was okay..."

As an adult and a parent, you often assume that you can rely on other adults and parents to have similar values as yourself. Obviously, this is not the case.

Some parents have double standards: "My daughter must be protected, but my son can sow wild oats." I remember one 13-year-old in a class when they'd all been complaining about parents who constantly worried about them getting raped, or pregnant, or AIDS.

She leaned back in her seat and said, "My dad says that if anything ever happened to me, he would die. Boy, I sure don't want my dad to die, so I am always really careful." Two boys spoke up and said, "You're really lucky, Corinne, but boys are supposed to be strong and take chances; girls are luckier, they're not." Out of the mouths of babes!

Other parents believe that teens should be allowed complete freedom: "They'll find out soon enough about making mistakes and have to clean up their own messes." The trouble with that philosophy is that their children may take your child down with them.

Many parents work hard at teaching their children to care for others, to respect others, but do not spend enough time teaching their own children to care for and respect themselves. Teens need help to extricate themselves from situations in which too much empathy for friends may mean putting themselves in danger.

I like to point out to all young people that nature makes our stomachs ache, our bowels feel loose, or our bladders feel full, "on purpose, as a defense," when we are very worried or scared. I tell them to pay attention to their bodies. "Sometimes your body will tell you that you are in danger before your head will."

You may want to rehearse dangerous situations with your young people. I suggest the dinner table as a good discussion site – that way the whole family can participate. You might be surprised at how wise a six-year-old can be about a teen problem.

Let's look at some typical situations; let's play the "What if" game.

"What would you do if your friend wanted to shoplift, to vandalize, to smoke a cigarette, to drink a beer, to joyride, to try drugs, to have sex?"

If your child doesn't come up with anything, suggest that they might say, "I've got a stomach ache, I think I'm going to be sick, I better go home." Or, "I have terrible cramps, I think I have diarrhea, I better go."

Of course they will laugh and think it is a big joke. I like to laugh with them and even encourage them to think about sillier phrases. But I also point out to them that even adults use these excuses – "I have to visit the restroom, I have to fix my makeup, I've got a migraine" – to get themselves out of dates from hell, conversations with offensive people, or away from harassment.

Some parents will remember how difficult it was to say "no" to a friend or a group of friends when they were young. No one wants to look like a "chicken" or a "geek." And yet kids can be empowered by this little piece of science: psychological studies have shown that it only takes one person, speaking against a group decision, to give a new direction to the group.

I truly believe that deep down, most children really appreciate having firm rules and guidelines to live by. I have had children and teens tell me (secretly, in confidence) that they are so glad that their parent is a clergyperson, a lawyer, a doctor, or a member of an ethnic minority, "because they won't let me do things that other kids have the freedom to do." Parents rarely hear these sighs of relief, or at least not until the child is grown-up and more mature. Other children and teens have said, "Jennifer or Satinder or Mayling are lucky; their parents are strict Chinese, or lawyers, or teachers, and they are not allowed to go to sleepovers, or to drink, or..."

Of course, I am not suggesting that your rules be ironclad and that you remain inflexible in every instance. Dialogue with your young people is the key here. It is always fruitful to let them talk first, but ask them to be specific about their request. Exactly who will be there, which adults are supervising, what are their telephone numbers, what hours of the day or night are we talking about, etc. Never hesitate to phone other parents and check the details that your child has supplied. And if you decide that your child may participate, make certain that there are escape routes that are safe. Finally, every parent's bottom line (I hope) would be, "Call me if you need me, and I promise I will not be mad!"

Contraceptive News for Teens

I know that some folks will not agree with me, but I believe that teens should be knowledgeable about condoms – which brands are best, how to use them properly, that it's okay to feel comfortable buying them – even if they will not necessarily be having sex. Both boys and girls need to be fully informed. I'd even go so far as to suggest that they buy some, read the directions thoroughly, and, if they are male, try them on in private, alone!

Parents and others may also disagree with me when it comes to how much teens need to know about all the other contraceptives. In part, I hesitate to spend a lot of time in class studying other methods of contraception because I usually have limited time with the students and I'd rather spend that time on thorough condom teaching rather than on implants, IUDs, sponges, and injections. Teens cannot afford many of these alternatives to the condom; they cost far too much and they are too intrusive for most young women. On top of all that, the alternatives offer no protection against STDs.

I also want both males and females to be fully informed about oral contraceptives, or the pill as most teens call it. First, it does absolutely nothing to protect against STDs. I'd like to repeat that 25 times! So many teens and adults have no understanding about this. I hear it over and over: "I don't have to worry about STDs, I'm on the pill," or "I don't have to worry about diseases, my girlfriend is on the pill." My reply to boys: "When she says, 'Don't worry, I'm on the pill,' *worry*, and *run* to the nearest condom!"

I try to impress upon the boys that they are not wearing the condom to protect her, "You're wearing it to protect yourself, from infections and fatherhood." Too many men are hauled into court for child maintenance, crying to the judge, "But she told me she was on the pill." In the judge's place, I would say, and I *do* say to teens, "It is your penis and you are in charge of where it goes and what it does. Don't send it out without a condom. (Some people call condoms required 'evening wear.') If you don't want to be a father, don't have sex, or double bag! Take every protection for yourself. Most STDs are curable; fatherhood takes at least 19 years."

Girls don't always get the essential information about the pill either. It must be taken every day, not once in a while. It must also be taken at the same time every day (within two hours). There are also over-the-counter medications that might interfere with the efficacy of the pill. We now talk about the five "A's" with teens: antihistamines, antacids, alcohol, analgesics, and even prescription antibiotics can interfere with the pill.

Boys need to hear this too so that they know not to trust the pill for their own protection.

Another consideration must be monogamy. Teens, too often out of their own immaturity in relationships, swear that they are virgins or monogamous. "Serial monogamy," or a string of partners, one at a time over months or years, is the same to your body as having multiple partners. Unless each and every sexual encounter is protected by a condom, your risk for STDs rises exponentially. Every sexual contact counts and denial and minimization don't keep one safe.

I say this to teens: "Take care of yourself and each other. Don't have sex if you or your partner is not ready. When in doubt, run. Abstinence is still the safest choice.

"If you are positive that both you and your partner can handle *any* consequence, then always use condoms, every single time."

In an eleventh grade class:

Teen 1: Can't the guy just pull out and not leave sperm behind?

Meg: Some people believe that.

Teen 2: Yeah, the guy says he'll only put it in your vagina for one minute. Then he takes it out and you're safe.

Meg: So why doesn't everyone use this method?

All the girls in one voice: Cause guys lie!

The Morning-After Pill (Emergency Contraception)

It is essential for teens and sexually active adults to know about the morning-after pill (MAP). It is four pills, not one, despite the popular name "pill."

If there has been an incident of unprotected intercourse, or the condom broke, then the woman or teenage girl can go to a doctor, a clinic, or the emergency room of a hospital and ask for the MAP.

She takes two pills immediately, and two more pills 12 hours later. The pills must be taken within 72 hours of the intercourse, but the sooner after intercourse they are taken, the more effective in preventing a pregnancy they will be. The failure rate is very, very small. If a girl does get pregnant despite taking the MAP, there is no evidence that the MAP will have any effect on an early pregnancy.

Keep in mind that the MAP contains a relatively high dose of hormones, so it should probably not be used instead of regular types of contraception. Anyone who *does* need the MAP will want to consider using extra protection in the future.

It should go without saying that all rape victims should be offered the MAP.

To be fair, a few people do not accept the MAP, because of their antiabortion views, and so there will be doctors and other medical practitioners who might refuse to dispense it. My view of ethical behavior in this instance would be that those folks who hold this view should refer the woman or girl to someone else. But be aware that some will not agree with me and will not refer. Keep looking until you find someone who will help you.

Coca-Cola, Standing Up, and Some Other Myths

Beware the myths! All those old tales and wild rumors about what will prevent pregnancy are still alive and thriving among teens.

In case you've forgotten, let me remind you what some of these myths are: If you stand up and have sex, the sperm will fall out. If you have sex in a Jacuzzi or a lake or a hot tub, the water will wash the sperm out. Or, a variation on the theme, you can sit in a bath later and let the bath water wash away the sperm.

Here's another one: If a female urinates after intercourse, she will pass the sperm and not get pregnant. It's amazing how many people (not just young people, but adults too) know nothing about sexual anatomy. They express amazement that females have three openings between their legs and they believe that women urinate out of their vaginas.

Here's some more: You're not in any danger the first time you have sex; the first time is free. You have to be menstruating to get pregnant. If you're on your period, you won't get pregnant, and on and on.

None of the above is true! I'm even hesitant to put these in my book, but believe me, I do it because I have to say it again and again. None of the above is true!

The cola myth is especially enduring. It is amazing how many boys still believe they can kill sperm by drinking cola (so many still have their digestive systems confused with their reproductive systems), or by soaking their penises in it. When I ask why they believe this nonsense, they say, "Cola dissolves tacks, therefore it must kill sperm." (It always seems strange to me that they're not afraid to soak their penises in something that dissolves nails.) It is true, the acid in cola drinks will sometimes attack metal. But sperm are not made of metal.

Teenagers want to believe in cola because it's cheap and easy to get. But here's the science. All five colas have been tested. Colas simply energize the sperm so that they're in there and doing their job even faster. Sperm have only one goal in life – to find the ovum (egg). They do this

Some people say you can pickle your penis by sticking it in cola. Is that true?

exceptionally well. They travel at lightning speed and are up into the uterus and heading for the ovum within seconds. Preventing this takes knowledge and practice, not cola.

STDs and Teens

Chapter 10 in this book focuses specifically and in greater detail on STDs. At this point, I'd simply like to remind you that you need to be prepared to talk about STDs, doctors' exams, and treatments with your teen, especially if you suspect that your teen is sexually active.

First, make certain that they have had their hepatitis B shots. Some students now get them as part of their school vaccination program. It only protects against hepatitis B, not any of the other strains of hepatitis which may also be passed with intimate contact. Other vaccines are becoming available for other types of hepatitis.

Second, make certain that they understand that any intimate contact with an infected person can be dangerous. Some educators and materials talk about "outercourse" as a way to express intimacy without risking pregnancy. Some define outercourse as any sexual activity that does not involve any type of intercourse: hugging, kissing, fondling, intimate dancing, massage are examples. Others define outercourse as anything other than vaginal intercourse (including anal sex, oral sex, and digital sex).

Can STD's be transmitted just as easily through oral sex as anal or vaginal?

You must be aware that infections can be passed during oral sex, anal sex, and digital sex. I know girls who have had severe toxic shock, and I know one who died after having digital sex, because her boyfriend's fingers were not clean.

Teens who choose to be sexually active are often in furtive positions without access to cleanliness or protection. And in many situations, teens are under the influence of drugs and/or alcohol. It is impossible to take care of yourself or your partner if you are drunk or stoned. Life does not cancel the problem because of poor planning or control. Sperm, bacteria, and viruses only know warm, human bodies. It is not who you are but what you do that gets you in trouble.

A very good book that provides details about STDs and contraceptives is *A New Prescription for Women's Health*, by Dr. Bernadine Healy (Viking, 1995).

A Word or Three about Viagra

Not long ago, I heard this very disturbing story from a mother. One day her 15-year-old daughter, who had just had a baby and was only three weeks postpartum, approached her and asked if she could get her some Viagra. Horrified, the mother asked, "Why in the world do you think you need Viagra?"

And so the story came out. The girl, having just had a baby, was not feeling particularly amorous or interested in resuming sexual activity with her boyfriend – much to his dismay. He thought that if she took Viagra, her libido would return!

So much attention has been paid to Viagra, on television newscasts and in articles in national newsmagazines and newspapers, that many people – teens and younger children included – have come to think of it as some kind of sexual wonder drug. Unfortunately, what teens and many adults hear is a lot of hype, and not much science information. Is it any wonder that such misunderstandings arise?

Let's sort out the facts.

Impotency (the inability to achieve or maintain an erection) is a common problem among older men. This fact alone allows you to talk about how elderly people also (surprise, surprise) enjoy sexual activity.

Does Viagra have any affects if women take it?

Can it have any harm on the relationship? ie: more of a sex life changes feelings?

Viagra is a medicine, in pill form, that helps impotent men have an erection. This second fact allows you to talk about the need to keep bodies as healthy as possible by avoiding smoking and other risky activities that threaten health. (Of course, not all impotency is caused by poor self-care.)

Viagra works by keeping extra blood in the penis so that an erection can be maintained long enough for an orgasm and ejaculation to occur. In other words, Viagra is a "mechanical" aid for a physical condition. Viagra does not work on one's mind, creating more desire for sex or lustful moments. Our libido or sex drive is in our heads, not in our genitals.

Parents need to foster critical thinking in their teens and younger children. Who is making the most money from the product and do the benefits outweigh the side effects, even deaths, that have been reported?

As always, our children need to work at staying healthy, making wise choices, and never having a need for Viagra.

Believe It or Not, Teens Want to Talk

There have been several studies done with teens and young adults, in several Western countries, asking, "Who would you most like to be able to talk with about sexual issues?" Overwhelmingly, teens have said "parents." They will even admit that they themselves are somewhat at fault when this communication doesn't happen:

"I'm scared to ask questions." They are afraid that their parents will "freak," or "be mad," or "ground me," or "never let me out again."

I must admit that when I had three teenagers I had to bite my tongue until the blood ran to keep from "freaking." Do some deep breathing, enjoy the jokes, never criticize their sources or their friends, talk, and most important, listen.

Teens want you to respect their stories and to "listen to the *whole* story before you freak." When the story involves a friend who has done something foolish or dangerous, try sympathy before judgment. Something like, "Oh, the poor kid, what could have happened?" "What will happen now?" Remember how great a compliment it is to you when your teen lets you in on his or her life. So many teens suffer from a lack of a significant adult in their lives, one who is there for them, one who listens.

They Inspire Us All

The lovely thing about teens is that, for those who have had good teaching and who have not been exploited or had abuse ignored, their optimism and joy about their future relationships and marriage is marvelous to behold. They are full of self-confidence, not afraid to ask questions; they carry a healthy curiosity to all their activities, and their expectations for fulfillment are contagious. They bring all the positive indicators from the previous levels into their sexually mature adult lives. They inspire us all.

Practical Tips

Even the most educated and open teen can use a more private method of learning to be sexually mature. Books can be very useful and I see no reason why a senior teen shouldn't be exposed to books about healthy adult sexuality. When you give a teen a book such as *The Male Body: What Every Man Should Know About His Sexual Health*, by A. Morgentaler, you are not saying, "Here you are, now go out and become sexually active." We all need time to become well-educated, to have a multitude of questions answered, and to internalize new information.

Adolescent Checklist

Your adolescent child needs to know

- everything the previous age groups have learned, plus;
- the proper use of contraceptive devices, and their potential failure;
- detailed information about STDs (see pages 177–187).

They should also be working to develop

- an understanding of intimate relationships;
- relationship skills;
- refusal skills;
- confidence when going to a doctor (see pages 189–196).

6

The Sexually Mature Adult

Could you explain hysterectomies

How can u tell if you have breast cancer?

what is a vasectomy?

If a man has a vasectomy and his sperms don't comme out, will his testicles get really Big?

I have three basic indicators of adult sexual maturity that I have developed out of my medical and science approach. There are several others, developed by psychologists and sociologists that are equally valid and which I'll mention at the end of the chapter.

My own list begins with the ability to be comfortable with our bodies and to do the examinations on ourselves that doctors expect us to do for ourselves. Many women are unable to examine their own breasts on a monthly basis. Perhaps they were abused or grew up in an otherwise nurturing home, but one that was very repressed about sexuality. Touching their breasts then becomes impossible; they feel dirty, narcissistic, even sinful.

Our whole society rarely talks about male breast cancer and sadly the survival rate among males with breast cancer is much lower than it is for women.

We never talk about testicular cancer either, and yet most victims now are in their teens and young adulthood. Can you imagine what happens when I try to teach teenage boys to examine their testicles? "Gross, Meg, you're such a pervert!" Even the cancer societies rarely distribute their booklets teaching testicular exams.

When I am in colleges and universities, students of all ages come to me after a presentation and say, "I feel so awful; I didn't know about any of this stuff. I had a lover a year or two ago. I found a lump in her breast, or on his testicles, and I was too embarrassed to say anything." If that lover doesn't examine his or her own self, or is too embarrassed to go to the doctor, their life could be in danger.

The second indicator of sexual maturity on my list is that there would be no exploitation or abuse in relationships.

There are many, many ways to exploit or allow yourself to be exploited. For example, here's a couple I hear about from young people: "I had to have sex with him; he gave me a ride home," or "She owed me sex; she invited me in for coffee."

But the issue of exploitation that worries those of us in the sexual health field the most is the kind of exploitation that takes place when two people do not talk to each other about STDs. They don't talk about sexual history, testing, or even protection. I often hear excuses such as, "I don't have to worry about STDs, my girlfriend is a nurse, my boyfriend is an accountant, I only sleep with people who drive BMWs," or my personal favorite, "I don't have to worry because I only go with people I meet at the most expensive night clubs!" A few more: "I'm only having sex with people at university," or "My friends introduced me to this person and they wouldn't introduce me to anyone with an infection." Unfortunately, bacteria and viruses don't know what kind of car you drive or in which nightclub you met this person. A sexually mature person would not be too shy, embarrassed, or drunk to protect their lives.

The third indicator is respect and understanding of society's laws, taboos, and boundaries around sexuality. No matter how much some people may know about sexuality, if they rape, abuse, or sexually harass, we would not call them sexually mature.

Hysterectomies and Vasectomies

Not surprisingly, young people aren't just aware of the changes happening to their own bodies, they are frequently aware that their parents are undergoing changes too. I often get questions about hysterectomies and vasectomies; children hear their parents discussing these things and come to me looking for information.

A hysterectomy is relatively easy to explain to children. First, they need to know about the uterus, of course. When you've explained that it is a muscular bag or pouch, about as big as four curled fingers, designed to hold the developing baby, then you can help the child to understand a woman can live without it.

There are several reasons for removing it and it is up to you as the parent to explain as much as you think is appropriate about the need for the surgery. The most important issue is to explain simply, at first, and allow the child to ask any questions. Remember that all that is truly important to children is that their parent or adult friend will be all right.

Vasectomies and tubal ligations are considered to permanent methods of birth control. Most children are curious about how they work. When the woman's fallopian tubes are "tied," the doctor usually removes a piece of each tube and ties off the ends. The ovum is still released from the ovary each month. It is pure protein, about the size of a grain of sand, and dissolves after a few hours. The woman still has menstruation and sexual intercourse is still possible. The sperm will dissolve in the uterus.

Vasectomies can be done in the doctor's office under a local anesthetic. The scrotum is opened with a small incision, the *vas deferens* are cut and tied off. Semen is still produced by the prostate gland and so the man may still have sex with the usual ejaculation, but after a few weeks there will not be any sperm in the semen. The testicles gradually stop producing sperm since it is impossible for them to leave the testicles. Remember that sperm are microscopic in size and that they are protein too, so they are easily absorbed by the man's body. The testicles do not enlarge.

Children also ask if the man still desires sex and it is good to explain that desire is in our heads so a vasectomy does nothing to change the man's interest in having sex.

Adult Sexuality and Change

Young people in today's world (and of course their parents too) are facing a new phenomenon in human history. The majority of first-time parents are now over the age of 30. Many parents are starting second families after divorce, or are in blended families in which one or both parents bring with them children from previous marriages. Quite often, the new marriage will also produce children. The situation then becomes quite complicated, with "your kids," "my kids," and "our kids" all needing appropriate attention. And then there are the older career-oriented women (and a few men) who have never married, but who have decide to "go it alone" and begin parenting.

All of this so-called "delayed parent-ing" means that by the time your children have finished puberty in their midteens, you yourself may be going through hormonal changes! Teens are not unaware that their parents are going through these changes and so I get a lot of questions about menopause. Sometimes I see teens who are really together, emotionally and physically quite mature, but their parents, their teachers, other relatives, or employers, are falling apart.

Please Explain What exactly Menopause is?

Male Menopause

Let's look at male menopause first. Other names for the male midlife changes have been coined: viropause, andropause, and male climacteric.

It is generally agreed in the medical field that there is a slow decline in testosterone production in men beginning in their early 40s. Unlike females, men do not ever cease production of "their" hormone entirely, but the diminishing testosterone levels can cause significant body changes. Most obvious is the "potbelly" of midlife, but there are other symptoms too. Unfortunately, to most male minds, these all involve loss. For example, men find that they have less energy, less intense erections, less hair, less patience, and get less sleep (as a result of more sleep disturbances). Some men try to overcompensate by driving themselves at work, at the gym, or in some other athletic endeavor. Some become restless sexually, and seek a younger woman's attention. Some feel driven to change jobs or to go back to university. Some men resort to alcohol or drugs, and some become increasingly violent in order to gain more control.

Try to imagine how all or any of these changes might affect a teenage son or daughter. Teens have told me about feeling puzzled, isolated, and uncared-for in the midst of these crises. Too many men carry all their worries inside, not talking, not acknowledging any of it. More tragically, too many make colossal decisions and changes without ever talking to their children or spouse, without consulting them or even recognizing the enormity of what they've done.

Perhaps the saddest is the man who leaves his first wife and his children, goes off with a much younger woman, and then finds after a few months or years that the younger wife is tired of "the old man." He then has nowhere to go because the first family has rejected him.

Imagine what all of this tells a teen about sexuality and relationships. At this age, their own sexual health can be vulnerable. Too often they are forced to turn to other teens for support and end up in great trouble.

Men and their doctors need to be better educated about midlife hormonal changes. Fortunately, more research is being done and testosterone patches and other treatments are being marketed. Above all, men must learn to be honest with their kids. Open up, talk to your teens about your own changing sexuality. Ask questions, consult, make truly mature decisions about life changes, and care for your teens first of all. Don't drive them into the arms of someone who can't help them half as much as you could if you really tried.

I would like to recommend two recent books that offer excellent information on males in midlife: *Male Menopause*, by Jed Diamond (Sourcebooks, 1997); and *Midlife Man: A Not So Threatening Guide to Health and Sex for Man at His Peak*, by Art Hister, M.D. (Greystone Books, 1998).

Female Menopause

Some women truly sail through their perimenopause (up to ten years before their menses stop) and into their menopause without any symptoms or noticeable distress. You never hear about these women, or they are said to be mythical.

The normal age for menstruation to stop is between 40 and 59. The average age is 51. However, it can be much earlier for women who smoke, who have had a hysterectomy, or for those who have had a tubal ligation.

Some women experience what they would label "mild" or "nuisance" symptoms in their perimenopause. Perhaps they experience increased irritability, fatigue, unexplainable aches and pains, night sweats, or increased sensitivity to changes in temperature. Most who call these symptoms "mild" report no real alteration in the way they live their lives.

Other women find they cannot carry on as usual. They feel quite debilitated by night sweats or joint pain. Some are extremely distressed by their emotional changes and other symptoms that they would call "serious."

Each woman must be allowed to name her own level of discomfort. No one else has the right to tell her that she is exaggerating or minimizing the symptoms. That having been said, I would urge every woman to seek natural remedies first, and then medical help, if she or those around her consider it necessary.

Perhaps a bigger problem than the actual physical changes taking place are the many stereotypes about women and menopause – most of them false and prejudicial – that women face. Ageism and sexism rear their ugly heads and women become anxious and preoccupied with their bodies and their appearance. Some fill any spare time with exercise classes; they diet constantly, and spend large sums on cosmetics and surgery.

Again, imagine the messages that come through to teens when this happens. Any kind of "ism" is a sign of a lazy mind. Don't get caught up in a preoccupation with yourself, denying your teens attention and time that they still need from you.

Try to be intentional about the kind of behavior you model for them. Make a study of female menopause, exercise your mind, learn to celebrate changes, become an informed consumer of any medical help that you may need, and again, don't drive your teens away and into vulnerable situations. Finally, don't be afraid to discuss with your teen your own changing sexuality.

Two good books for women at midlife are *Facing Changes, Making Choices, Finding Freedom: Voices of Canadian Women at Mid-Life*, by Marilyn McCrimmon and Rosemary Neering (Whitecap, 1996); and *Mind Your Body: A Sexual Health and Wellness Guide for Women*, by Beth Howard (St. Martin's Griffin, 1998).

Are You a Sexually Mature Adult?

By now you'll have caught on to the idea that being an adult and being sexually mature don't necessarily go hand-in-hand. But where do you stand, personally?

At the beginning of this section, I outlined my own yardstick for gauging sexual maturity. The box, below, contains some other indicators which psychologists and sociologists use to gauge sexual maturity.

Of course, the fact the you're even reading this book should indicate that you're well on your way to full sexual maturity. Think about it. If you saw this book and couldn't stop laughing and making off-color jokes about it, you'd be stuck at the bathroom humor stage. If you were embarrassed or disgusted by the book, you'd be at the intermediate level. And if you told yourself that you didn't need this, you knew it all, you'd be at the adolescent level.

So give yourself a pat on the back and carry on an ever vigilant quest for more information. And don't be afraid to grab every teachable moment to help your children grow along with you.

Adult
Checklist

1. Sexually mature people are able to participate fully and joyfully in a sexual relationship, with mutual regard and respect, but they can be alone too. They do not need sex to feel complete.

2. Sexually mature people accept their gender, orientation, and status in society with confidence and satisfaction. They are not bitter or predatory.

3. Because sexually mature adults have the above two indicators and are secure themselves, they can nurture and actively encourage everyone else in their community.

7

Alternate Ways to Get Pregnant

How does a test tube baby be made?

Is it posible for a girl to get pregnet with out intercourse.

In a spermbank, how do the men take out the sperm from their body.

Do you have to have sex to have a baby.

My English mother-in-law was a wonderful person who supported me as a daughter-in-law and as an independent woman from the very first moment she met me. I had met my husband, her son, in Philadelphia, where we both worked, but then we went to live in England. I was often intimidated by the culture, by the professors my husband taught with, and by their families. But my mother-in-law would always say, "You must always remember that we were all got and came the same way." That was the early 1960s. Times have changed.

Actually, some alternative methods of conception are almost as old as humans. The Bible certainly talks about sisters having babies for sisters. Many ancient and not-so-ancient cultures and faiths made male adults responsible for all the children and women in their extended families. If a man's brother died, he was to take on the care of the widowed sister-in-law and sometimes he was to inseminate her to keep her and the children in the family.

When we hear stories of babies being conceived by artificial insemination and with turkey basters, we can guess that humans probably figured out how to do that hundreds, if not thousands, of years before turkey basters were invented.

At the present time, children can be conceived by a variety of methods, some involving doctors and hospitals, some not.

When I talk to youngsters, especially the last few years, I find that most children know something about test-tube babies, surrogate mothers, and artificial insemination. They hear about these things on television, they read about them (often in the more sensational newspapers), and they talk about them with each other. In almost every school there are also some children who are fully aware that they were not created during sexual intercourse; they have all

If someone is a lesbian how could they get a baby?

the details of their conceptions and are more than willing to share the information.

Sperm Banks

One point of clarification that children seem to need is how sperm banks work. They all seem to imagine that sperm banks are located in every community and that they operate like the Bank of America, or food banks. Anyone can walk in and be a donor, or walk in and make a withdrawal.

It is good to explain that sperm banks are few and far between and that they are often located in big university hospitals, to which only specialist doctors have access. And they don't look like The Bank of America; they're round, steel, freezing cylinders, perhaps as big as an oil drum. That's it, nothing fancy, not an architectural marvel.

What do they do at a sperm bank?

Test-Tube Babies

Another very real misunderstanding is created in children's minds by the media's use of the term "test-tube babies." First, sperm and ovum are not in a test tube – ever! Doctors usually use glass saucers called petri dishes. Second, the sperm and ovum are in the petri dishes, in a special incubator, for hours, not weeks. (The scientific name for the process is "*in vitro* fertilization.") Once the ovum is fertilized, joined by the sperm, the ovum is placed in the woman's uterus, by the doctor, through her vagina. After that, hopefully,

Can you pass a egg from your own body into another women's body?

it develops as a normal pregnancy would. The baby is not growing in a test tube!

Honesty

Since so many parents now share their conception trials, errors, and successes with their adult friends and relations, as well as with their children, it seems prudent to be honest here.

These days, all parents should be prepared to have their children ask questions and tell stories about the details they hear. When a child comes home from school and says that Billy's mom is pregnant, in the best possible world it truly would be no one's business how it happened. A mature and responsible parent would not pry or allow their child to gossip, even if you have personal details about Billy's mom, or dad, that would suggest that the usual conception was not possible. I'd like to repeat this. It is no one's business! It is personal, and if Billy's mom chooses not to share, that is her prerogative. Rejoice in the new life!

Curiosity is normal, of course, and if your child asks questions such as, "How can she have a baby if she doesn't have a husband?" then you could explain how it is possible for this to happen in general, but not how it happened for your neighbor specifically.

Please don't forget to teach good manners and the need to respect boundaries. Perhaps you could add that it wouldn't be polite to go to school and share all this information with the other students. Praise your child's questions, but expect good manners in return.

Now, some bigger questions arise. Should you tell your own children how they

In a third grade classroom, a teacher introduced me, explained that I would be teaching about bodies, and said, "Put up your hand whenever you have a question."

One little girl immediately shot up her hand and asked, "Does a lady have to have a husband to have a baby?"

Before I could open my mouth to answer her, a boy shouted out, "Of course she does. He has to drive her to the hospital!"

were conceived? When should you tell them? How many others do you tell and how do you tell them?

Years ago, adoption was shrouded in very tight secrecy. Since then, we've learned how damaging this practice was. Now, no one hides adoption and we've matured tremendously around that issue.

But we are still pioneering alternative conceptions, plus the whole concept of how to tell the children of these conceptions. I don't think that there are any absolute answers to the above questions – yet. But I would like to suggest that family secrets are not a good idea. From all the personal stories that people have shared with me, my impression is that it is best to be honest with your child as early in his or her life as possible.

If you remember the stages, preschoolers accept the information like little scientists – no emotional baggage, just the facts. If you told your three- or four-year-old that a stork brought them, or that Daddy got them at Sears on sale, they'd accept the lie in exactly the same way they would accept the truth. So why lie or evade the questions?

Primary children are easy, too, because of their mechanical curiosity. Their little engineers' minds kick in and they are very accepting of factual information. Don't let any of your own emotional baggage influence your presentation. "Just the facts, sir, just the facts," as the detectives used to say.

do kids relly come from the stork

If you wait until they are intermediates to tell them, they often feel betrayed: "Why didn't you tell me before?" or outraged that their life to date now seems like a lie. Or they are so shocked and embarrassed that they don't ask the questions that will plague them for years.

Of course, children often overhear family gossip, or someone secretly tells the story, or neighborhood rumors reach the ears of the school age child. If you want to be the first to tell your child, be certain that you are indeed the first, not the neighbors.

What to tell them is another question with no absolute answer. Basic information is fine to start. Perhaps something such as, "Daddy didn't have quite enough sperm and so a doctor helped us and we got some sperm from a donor to make you," or "I wanted to have a child, but I didn't have a husband, so a doctor helped me, and another man gave us some of his sperm."

You may want to explain that when there is a donor for the sperm, the rules say that he cannot be identified. You can still, however, celebrate the man's generosity.

If you know the donor of the sperm or ovum, hopefully the two biological parents have agreed before the insemination that the child will be told, whether the donor or the surrogate are to be present in the child's life or not. I have heard many, many different stories from parents about who the donor was: a friend (gay or straight), a relative, or a relative stranger, an acquaintance chosen for their physical attributes, or whatever. My best advice is to be honest, but be prepared to support your child if and when the story is to be told in the community.

Children cannot be expected to maintain their confidence forever, without wavering in the face of thoughtless and cruel remarks, especially from other children. There will always be people who are uneducated and self-centered with their own curiosity, and who ask questions. Show your child how courageous and mature you can be and they will be able to model themselves after you.

Finally, there are beginning to be resources to help parents explain alternate conceptions to children. The medical center that specializes in helping infertile couples may have material, so be sure to ask.

One book that I recommend highly is written by Holly H. Smith and is called *I Was Created by Love and Donor Insemination*. It is beautifully written for children of any age, and has delightful illustrations. Ask your local bookstore to order it or contact Holly yourself in Ladysmith, BC, Canada, by fax at (250) 245-2106, or by e-mail at holly@island.net.

PART TWO

Straight Answers to
the Questions
Your Children
Will Ask

8

Straight Answers to the Questions Your Children Will Ask

Anon- why do people always find it OK to look at girl's naked bodys but it's not OK to look at boy's naked bodies?

How do gay men make love?

what is oral sex?

IS MASTERBATING BAD FOR YOU?

How often does an average couple have sex.

I don't believe that there is one "right" answer that a parent must give when their child or teenager asks a personal question. Much depends on the age of the child and on the comfort level of the parent.

Children and teens today ask questions that we would *never* have asked our parents; the fear of our parents' wrath would have kept us silent even though we may have wondered about the same things.

Take the questions as compliments. Remember: they wouldn't ask if they truly expected you to be upset. First, return the compliment: "I'm glad that you felt comfortable asking me that question and I am not mad at you, but I might need a little time to think, so just hang on a moment while I sort out a good answer for you."

Let's look at some common personal questions that children and teens might ask.

"What's a Virgin?"

You might begin by gently and casually asking, "Where did you hear the word?" or "What do you think it means?" Never laugh at or tease your own child's misunderstandings.

A good answer would be, "A virgin is someone who has never had sex."

If there has been teasing about who is a virgin or not at school, then you can point out how unkind this is and how those who are participating may not have the courage that your

---

Fourth grade boy at Discovery School: I looked up sex in the dictionary at home.

Meg: Oh, good.

Boy: Then I looked it up in the school dictionary and it was there too!

*are you a pevert
if you look up
sexual words
in the
Dictonary*

child has to ask questions at home.

Sometimes I hear about a teacher or a principal who overreacts to this kind of teasing in the school or on the playground. The most mature educator would understand children's curiosity and misunderstanding around these issues.

A healthy way to deal with it would be to calmly and briefly explain to the whole class or group that there is a scientific description of this word in any dictionary. Read the definition aloud and then explain that the behavior they have been exhibiting is inappropriate. Now that they have thought about it "like scientists" they do not have to repeat the behavior. Period!

"Do You and Mom (Dad) Still Have Sex?"

Please don't forget to celebrate sexual activity in a healthy marriage. Don't hide the fact that you and your partner have sex. Children need to know that parents who love each other love to have sex.

I meet so many children who have a pretty good idea that their parents have sex - still. They've crept downstairs and seen amorous activity taking place on the couch, or they've heard noises in the night, or crept upstairs from the television room on Saturday morning. (Isn't that why they invented Saturday morning cartoons?) They are filled with anxiety when they tell me about it: "Why are they doing that, aren't they too old, are they perverts?" When I tell them how lucky they are to have parents who love each other and that I hope they'll love each other and have sex forever, all

Is there sex after marriage? Is there sex after 50?

My parents are over 40 & have sex all the time is it criminal?

I think so

that anxiety vanishes and huge smiles of relief and pride break out on their faces.

Of course, I also say, "Some boys and girls have moms and dads who are divorced or separated and they don't have sex anymore. But most moms and dads hope that one day they will have someone else to love and have sex with because most adults think that having sex with someone you love is a wonderful thing." That comforts the children in the class who have single parents who may or may not be seeing someone new.

I have tried to make this last statement free of heterosexism too, because there are growing numbers of children who are doing their best to cope with parents in homosexual unions. The homophobia in some communities is a crushing burden for children to bear.

When young children hear about sexual intercourse, many say, "Wow, will you call me the next time you and Dad do that?" Most parents would say "no" without thinking for a second, and that is appropriate. Go on to explain that their curiosity is normal, but that having sex is private. You might like to remember your sense of humor and add, "When you are married, I won't ask about your lovemaking either."

"Do You and Dad Do Oral Sex?"
"How Many People Have You Frenched?"
"Were You a Virgin When You Got Married?"

Much depends here on your sense of privacy. Here are some things to consider. Children come with an uncanny ability to detect lies, so don't lie. You may wish to say, "I'd rather not talk about my personal sex life. When you are an adult, I promise not to ask about yours." But acknowledge the naturalness of his or her curiosity: "I'm not mad at you for asking. I wondered about my parents

Is Oral sex O.K.?

too when I was your age, but I think it is private."

Other parents may want to say something about their sexual activities before or after they married. Perhaps something like this: "No, I wasn't a virgin when we got married, but it was a different world back then (when the Earth was cooling). We didn't know about AIDS or chlamydia; now we know that there are life-threatening STDs that often have no symptoms, and I think we'd better talk about this some more."

You might want to talk about how television and movies suggest that a young person is a nerd or a loser if they're not having sex, but rarely do they talk about emotional involvement. How many of those first-time partners remain together? Girls constantly talk about being dumped by the boy once they've agreed to have sex. The old adage, "Boys give love to get sex, and girls give sex to get love" is still alive.

Go gently into these conversations with young teens. It is possible that they are asking because they themselves have been exploited (when drunk at a party) by someone, or have a friend who has been.

Often, children are not asking about your personal life at all. The *real* question is, "Is it all right to French kiss," "Is it safe to have sex at my age," "Can you talk to me honestly about oral sex?"

In every movie the have sex. Why don't the star have a baby?

Can Paraplegics Have Sex?

This question comes up for people of all ages whenever disabled people or events for disabled people make the news. In recent times, we have only to think of the tragic accident involving Christopher Reeves (Superman), the Terry Fox Run, or the Man in Motion Tour. Adults don't generally voice their questions, but children do.

Some severely disabled persons have full sexual functions and are capable (with assistance) of having sex and reproducing. Some people who are disabled cannot.

I like to respect the child's question; their curiosity is normal. I will explain that much depends on the nature of the injury or deformity. You cannot tell by simply looking at the person who is in a wheelchair or on crutches, or who walks with an obvious disability. Doctors and nurses may be able to help disabled persons overcome their physical limitations and enable them to have sex or babies.

I also point out, however, that although I am pleased that they felt confident enough to ask me (the sex teacher), it would not be polite to ask the disabled person. Encourage empathy: "You wouldn't like to be asked such a personal question either, would you?"

What's an Orgasm?

A male orgasm is easy to explain. You might try this: "A male has an orgasm when his penis gets erect and sperm and semen are ejaculated from his penis. It makes him feel very good and then his penis relaxes and he feels relaxed too."

It is much harder to explain a female orgasm, mainly because you can't focus on an ejaculation, although some women will feel very wet and some may experience a kind of ejaculation of vaginal fluid.

Several books attempt to explain the female orgasm to children by associating it with the increasing tension you feel when you are about to sneeze. Finally, there is a release of that tension when you sneeze. I like to add, "But an orgasm feels a million times better than a sneeze."

Why do people make noise when they have sex?

One caution I'd like to suggest for parents is around noises and orgasms. Far too many children and teens are exposed to television and movie makers' stereotypes of human orgasms. In these ridiculous portrayals, there is a lot of noise, there are moans, heavy breathing, sweating, groaning, shouting, even screaming. I have had children ask me, "Why does the lady scream when you do it to her?" "Why do people moan?" and even, "Why do you have to beat the lady before you do it?"

Please consider talking to your children about these images and how the movie makers exaggerate simply to fascinate viewers. Even some adults think that they must behave in the same way and so they shout and scream because they think they should. It is sad how many people believe the Hollywood version to be the norm.

Talk to your young people about what lovemaking is like for sexually mature and healthy adults. It is not a competition, it is not a marathon, and it doesn't require Academy Award-winning performances.

> On movies I saw a man sucking on a girl's boobs. The girl was moaning alot but when I did that to my girlfriend she didn't make a sound. Why?

"What Does Gay, Lezy Mean?"
"How Do They 'Do It'?"
"Why Are People Gay?"

Once upon a time in human history, babies who were born as twins or triplets were killed because they were considered bad luck. Children who were born left-handed were beaten or killed because it was believed that they were possessed by Satan. Children who had red hair or retained their blue eyes after birth were abandoned as "devils."

We now believe that all of the above is superstitious nonsense and we've matured to understand that about 10 percent of any population will be born left-handed, blue-eyed, or as part of a multiple birth.

I do not believe that it is useful to belabor the question of why people are gay. A parent's best response, at first, might be, "No one knows exactly why some people are homosexual, just as no one knows why some people are left-handed." Every single person is human first.

It might be helpful to add that people used to believe it was "caused" by something that happened to a child, such as an absent father, not enough hormones, or abuse. Now we know that homosexuality is not something you can "catch," and that many gays and some lesbians feel that they were born with their orientation already in place. Some people may choose to live in a homosexual partnership and/or community because of their experiences of abuse or isolation or whatever.

The main point that I hope parents would consider making is that every one of us is allowed to call ourselves whatever we like. No one has the right to call us names or to discriminate against us because of our orientation, race, religion, or anything else.

how can you tell if someones gay

My response, once I have honored the student's right to ask the question, "Why are people gay?" and have explored the issue with them briefly, is to ask, "Who cares why they are gay? What any of us do in our bedroom is private."

I want to acknowledge their natural curiosity, but I also want to teach good manners. I want justice for everyone and I want no more suicides over worries about orientation. As one teen said, "Why would I *choose* to be gay in a straight world? My risks for STDs, suicide, drug and alcohol are higher than in any other group. I didn't choose. I just *am!*"

My dream is that, one day soon, we, as humans, will be able to drag ourselves into a greater maturity about those who are born with a homosexual or bisexual orientation. I say "soon" because homophobia is killing our kids, no matter what their orientation. Suicides, among teens and young adults, are often related to fears around orientation – fears that are exacerbated by homophobic putdowns, bashings, jokes, and rantings by public figures. Testicular cancer rates are rising among teens and young men who are afraid to examine themselves: "It means I'm gay if I touch myself."

Too many teens are trying to prove that they are real men or women and heterosexual by engaging in sexual intercourse or by becoming pregnant long before they are ready for those responsibilities.

The younger the child is when parents answer the above questions, the more the child takes the information "like a scientist," without prejudice. Here is one way to answer a younger child's questions: "Some people are only interested in making love to someone of the opposite sex when they are grown-up, and some people, when they are grown-up, will only be interested in making love to people of their own sex. A gay man would like to be in love with another gay man, and a lesbian woman would only be interested in making love with another lesbian woman."

Primary children will normally shrug their shoulders and ask "What's for lunch?" after this explanation. Older children will commonly ask, "But what do they do?" I have had 85-year-old people ask me that question! Here's one possible answer: "There are four ways to have sex and homosexuals have sex the same ways that heterosexuals have sex. One way is

How do gays and lesbians have sex?

vaginal sex; another way is oral sex; then there's anal sex, and finally digital sex. A large proportion of gay men only have oral sex, some enjoy anal sex, but large numbers of heterosexual partners use anal sex, too.

Of course, fingers get put into vaginas and children in elementary school do a lot of gossiping about "fingering."

Most children will respond with "Ooh gross" when you tell them about each of the four ways to have sex. A good response might be, "I'm glad you think it is gross at your age; children are not supposed to have sex. But even when you are a grownup, you never have to do any of those activities if you don't want to do them. *Whoever says 'no,' rules!* "

For teens and children beyond the age of seven or eight, it would also be good to point out that although a woman can't get pregnant unless sperm go into the vagina, anyone can get STDs growing in their mouth, throat, eyes, anus, or vagina, and these can cause serious life-threatening infections. It is heartbreaking when young people think that only gays can get AIDS during anal sex, not heterosexuals; or that venereal warts will only grown on genital tissue; or that toxic shock syndrome is only from tampons. Most STDs will flourish on any mucous membrane anywhere in the body, and the bacteria do not know or care about the person's orientation. They simply recognize warm, moist, human bodies.

An 11-year-old once asked his parents, "What do gay men do that moms and dads don't do, that gets them into trouble with STDs and AIDS?"

The parents answered, "Nothing. Both gay and straight people get into trouble if they have unprotected intercourse, no matter what kind."

If you are having a sexual relationship with someone of the same sex canyou get s.t.d's

A teachable moment might include an opportunity to talk about what your teen might do if he or she is anxious or afraid of being propositioned by a gay or lesbian friend or acquaintance.

You could begin by discussing with your child how difficult it must be for people who are homosexual, in our homophobic society, to come out openly about their orientation. If that was possible, then the field of potential partners would be obvious.

Given that many persons are not "out," it is possible that approaches may be made to people who are heterosexual. You could advise your teen or young adult to respond in exactly the same way they would if a heterosexual person approached them: "I'm sorry, but I am not interested in a sexual relationship." They may want to add, "I really like you and I want to continue to be friends, but I am heterosexual."

Some teens worry that if they have been approached (or abused) by a person of the same sex, it must mean that they are homosexual. I often hear, "What did they see in me that would suggest that I am gay or lesbian? Am I doing something wrong, giving off the wrong vibes? Do they know something secret about me that I don't know myself? What if I feel erotic feelings about a same sex friend, teacher, or youth leader?"

I think that it is interesting that two of my personal friends have told me about similar moments of comfort being given when they were anxious teenagers. Both were enormously troubled by thoughts that they might be gay. They both were at summer camps run by their religious affiliations and both finally confided their

I think I'm lesbeen but I Kind of like guys what should I do?

is it weird if I don't find girls attractive at my age?

worries to counselors, one a Christian clergyperson and the other a Jewish rabbi. Both counselors replied to these teens with a musing, thoughtful tone: "Yes, I understand your worries. I think that every teen has those same worries." That was all either of the men said, but both boys reported feeling enormous relief and an end to their angst.

Even more interesting, one of my friends is heterosexual and the other friend is gay.

WHAT IF YOU KNEW SOMEONE, WHO WAS GAY? CAN YOU STILL BE THEIR FRIEND? CAN YOU TELL THEM YOU DON'T LIKE GAYS?

Sometimes all we need is to know that we are "normal," whatever that means! Teens especially need this reassurance and it can be life-saving to suggest patience (time will help to sort out these questions) and that the feelings are perfectly normal in adolescents.

One last word for parents and our whole community to consider: We have come a long way in human history. We no longer tolerate racist name calling or sexist name calling. I think that it is time to get tough about name calling around orientation. In today's classrooms and on today's playgrounds, sports fields, and arenas, if one child used a racial slur against another child, he'd be hauled on the carpet so fast his head would spin. It is time to do the same when confronted with other hateful names.

Sadly, I've heard adults excuse this behavior because, "he doesn't know what he is saying." That is the coward's way out. Get brave, be mature, grow up, and put a stop to it! We are all injured by name calling. Our children need *peace* and *respect* to be healthy – and so do adults.

Is Masturbating Bad for You?

First, some scientific facts. All babies are born with the ability to have an orgasm. Babies touch their genitals long before they are born. A boy's penis begins to get erections 17 weeks into the pregnancy. We are all born sexual beings. If it was bad for us, nature would have made our arms shorter!

Some children exhibit a great deal of interest in their genitals, others never give parents any hint of interest. It is normal to masturbate and it is normal not to masturbate. (Males cannot run out of sperm; the testicles make sperm constantly.) Thank goodness we know that now!

The message that needs to be given to children as soon as you can talk and reason with them is that touching themselves is private. "I know it feels good, but you need to do that in the bedroom by yourself." You want to give them positive messages about their bodies, but you also want to protect them from abuse.

Let's imagine a scenario with an immature babysitter. If you allow your child to masturbate when they are watching television, while you're reading them a story, or in "public," the babysitter can say, "Hey, that looks interesting. Let me show you how I do it," and the child can be drawn into an abusive situation.

Many parents these days no longer punish children for touching themselves, but they don't say anything either. Unfortunately, that leaves children open to abuse. So much of what we teach our

Will masturbating damage my genitals?

After you have sex will the sperm grow back?

children about sexual health is about good manners, and touching genitals is private.

What about Nudity in the Home?

This isn't a question kids usually ask, but it's certainly a common question I get from parents. Specifically, parents want to know about nudity in the home: how much is "normal"; when should parents and children, or siblings, stop bathing together; what should the guidelines be?

Many parents enjoy bathing with their children and most siblings love to bath together, especially in the preschool and early primary years. The general wisdom these days is to enjoy it while it lasts, because it won't last forever! Sometimes, it is the parent who begins to feel uncomfortable or simply crowded out as the children grow bigger. That is the time for the parent to say, "I'd like to have my bath or shower alone from now on. I need my privacy." That would be quite marvelous modeling by the parent. It gives the child permission to say the same thing when it becomes important for him or her to have privacy.

The situation would be the same for siblings who have enjoyed sharing a bath. When one says, "I don't want to do this anymore," or "I want to bath by myself tonight," that child rules. It is most important that the parent be there for the child and show respect for that child's developing boundaries. Sometimes a younger child will become shy before an older one does, or will want privacy one day, but not another day. They are

We are a family which spends a lot of time nude in the bathroom together Do you forsee any problems In the near future?

not testing their parents, they are testing themselves and their own boundaries. They need parents to respect that. Remember the cardinal rule: Whoever says "no," rules.

The Hard Questions

Always try to remind yourself when your child asks a hard question or makes a shocking statement that it is a fine compliment to you. If they truly thought that you were going to kill them, they'd never say anything. So stay calm, breathe, and keep your voice neutral. Try your best not to be angry, because that is what children fear most.

Give some basic factual answer and watch for their reaction. Do they need more information? Are they still there, looking at you expectantly? Are they nodding and saying, "That's what I thought," or "That's what my friend told me." Is there an obvious need for you to say more? If you don't know what else to say, say that. Give yourself time by promising that you'll find out more and tell them tonight or tomorrow. Be honest about your embarrassment or ignorance.

You might want to say something like this: "I am really proud of you for asking me this; my parents would have washed my mouth out with soap and I'd have been grounded for a year. I am not sure how to answer your question, but I will do my best. Can we talk more about this at bedtime? I am not mad at you and I want you to have a good answer; I just need some time to think or to find out what you should know."

What's a Blow Job, a B.J., a 69er? What Is Oral Sex, Anal Sex, Fingering?

Parents who are unaware of the exposure that even very young children have to these topics can be shocked by these questions. They will be especially upset when the

What is a blowjob

child uses company at the dinner table to shield themselves when asking these questions.

It is perfectly all right to say, "That is a good question, my dear, but not at the Christmas dinner table. We'll talk about it at bedtime." I warn you, though, that if you have normal friends and relatives, they will all want to stay for bedtime to hear your answer!

First, as always, remember that their question is a compliment; they trust you to give an honest answer. Second, don't be put off by your immature friend who suggests that you wash your child's mouth out with soap. Honor the question and the courage or self-esteem it took to ask the question.

Third, bless the time you've been given to think about what you want to say. You could dig out a dictionary and use that as a discussion starter.

Fourth, give them science and health information. Begin with scientific vocabulary if they have used slang or vulgarities.

"Oral sex is when two grownups are making love and they put their mouths on each other's genitals."

You know what your child's response will be. "Oh gross." Follow that with, "You never have to do that when you are grown-up if you don't want to. You rule!"

"Anal sex is when two grownups are making love and one puts his penis in his partner's anus. Sometimes gay men do that, and sometimes men do that with women." Again, whoever says "no," rules.

"Fingering is when fingers go into the vagina or anus."

Now it is important to give health information. First, if fingers are inserted into the anus, they should not later be inserted into the vagina because this can give the woman an infection.

Second, sperm must enter the vagina to create a baby. Remember that laughter often eases tension and allows or encourages integration of information. So you might point out that if sperm are swallowed or placed in the anus, they will come out as "poo" or stool. If you happen to be dealing with primary age children (ages five to eight), you're back to their favorite subject and gales of laughter will follow.

But, and it is a big BUT, if one or both partners have an infection, the bacteria or virus can be transferred from the genitals or fingers, anus or mouth, to the other person. Most bacteria and viruses will grow wherever there is a mucous membrane. So it is possible to have STDs growing in the throat, mouth, eyes, anus, and any part of the genitals.

Impress upon your child or teen the importance of regular medical testing and being honest with the doctor about which sexual activities have been practiced.

I ask teens to ask themselves, "Can I go to the doctor with comfort? Can I be honest with my doctor about my sexual activities?" And most important, "Could I tell my partner if I had an infection?" If their answer is an agonized, "Oh no, I'd rather die," then I suggest that they're not ready for a sexual relationship. There are many adults who should be asking themselves these questions too.

What about Pornography?

You may find pornographic pictures, magazines, or videos in your child's possession, or they may ask you about pornography because they've heard about it or seen it somewhere.

Above all, keep calm in front of your child. You could begin by acknowledging a natural curiosity: Why do people make these pictures? Who are these people? Why would anyone buy or rent pornography?

You might explain that some people don't get a chance to learn about nude bodies and healthy sexuality from their parents or their schools and so they look at pornography.

It seems important to me to explain that people would not take part in the industry if they were not being paid a lot

why do people make porno?

of money or being forced to participate with drugs and/or violence. The pornography industry is riddled with exploitation and children need to understand that the smiles, noises, and actions are acting, not real life. These are not sex-mad people who are enjoying themselves. Unfortunately, AIDS and suicides are common in the business.

Don't hesitate to point out to children and teens that the glossy pornography magazines also portray unrealistic body images. No one looks that good in real life; they use plastic surgery, makeup, special lighting, and airbrush the images of both males and females.

Don't forget to tell your children that no one is allowed to take their picture, clothed or not, without your permission. Some abusers who exploit children by photographing them for pornography will claim innocence: "I never laid a hand on them." What a load of denial! It is clearly against the law in almost every jurisdiction to photograph children for sexual exploitation.

Always be prepared to talk about the illegal or deviant activities that they may see: sex with children, animals, weird impossible positions, sadism, bondage, and so on. Some children have told me that because they saw "it" in a magazine or on a video, it must be okay.

You also want to stress that two people must agree to any activity. It is against the law to force anyone, and very bad manners to try to persuade someone, if they don't want to do it. Again, whoever says "no" in a sexual relationship, rules. I tell children, "No matter how curious you may be or how much you want to try something, if the other person does not agree, you are out of luck! Don't put yourself in danger by insisting."

I was once asked to be an expert

Is pornography real

Can you get pregnant from sex with animals.

witness when a teenager was charged with sexual assault. The story was that when he and his girlfriend were "making out," he had put his fingers in her vagina. She said "no" twice, and after the second time, he didn't repeat the action. The rest of the evening the date seemed to go well; she didn't say anything about the incident, they went out for burgers and he took her home.

She then called her girlfriend to talk about the date and her friend's mother overheard the story. This woman then told the girl's mother and the charges were laid.

Often, when I share that story with young people, the boys will say, "Oh yeah, Meg, what are we supposed to do then? Are we supposed to stop everything and say, 'Excuse me, Dear, may I put my fingers in your vagina?'"

At this point, I don't usually have to reply, the girls in the room do, and loudly: "Yes!"

The message here is that you must be able to talk to your partner about your boundaries and theirs. If you can't talk about these issues *before* you begin any lovemaking, then you are not ready for sex. And that is a good thing to know about yourself.

If you can reassure the child who is interested in pornography that you understand their curiosity but that you understand their curiosity but that there are other books and videos to look at that satisfy our curiosity in more healthy, non-exploitative ways, the child will probably reject the pornography.

One question we as adults should be asking is, "Why can a child or teen see the most degrading pornography in corner stores and on adult video store windows, but not go to their church, school, or public library and take out books about healthy sexuality?" It seems odd that many adults resist making sexual health manuals

IN LOTS OF MAGAZINES LIKE COSMOPOLITAN PEAPLE WRITE SEXUAL FANTASIES. WHY DO THEY DO THIS.

and videos available in public libraries, but do nothing about the proliferation of pornography.

Finally, don't be afraid to talk to your children about the more subtle pornography that is used in television and magazine advertising and on music videos. Practice critical viewing skills aloud with your family.

One family I know mutes the commercials and plays a game called, "What are they selling, and how are they selling it?" The children picked up very quickly that if they bought product X, they would also get beautiful tanned bodies, fast cars, and hot women/men.

Encourage them to develop their discernment and even to call or write to protest when they are offended. Exploitation puts everyone at risk and sometimes one voice can put healthy attitudes back into our communities.

What's a Prostitute?

Children hear about prostitution on the news, on television, and in movies all the time, but they often believe that prostitutes are nymphomaniacs and will be eager to have sex with anyone who passes by.

You might explain that prostitutes are much more interested in getting money. In most jurisdictions, selling and buying sex is illegal. Unfortunately, some people think that they have no options but to buy or sell sex. Assure your children that they will have lots of healthy, safe choices when they are adults, and they won't ever have to be on the streets in such an unsafe way.

How come some people sell sex? Isn't it a dirty job?

What should kids do if a hooker asks you to do sex?

What Is Cross-Dressing? What Is a Transsexual?
What Is a Transvestite? What's Drag?
How Do You Get a Sex Change?

Afternoon talk shows are very popular and even if your child does not watch them, they will hear about them from those who do. Music videos also bring out many of these questions with their portrayals of cross-dressing and the like, all designed to titillate and exploit everyone's natural curiosities.

I believe that the best answers to these questions include science and health information. Be as honest as you can be.

One of the reasons that these topics fascinate youngsters and adults is because they don't know the facts and their curiosity is stimulated when the issues are taboo.

Help your child or teen sort out the scientific words. A transsexual or a transgendered person is one who believes, from a very early age, that he or she is in the wrong body. These people should not be confused with homosexuals or cross-dressers. Transgendered people are those who earnestly desire sex-change therapy and surgery as adults.

Children are full of questions about why someone would want to have a sex change.

In my experience, one of the anxieties behind these questions is tied to their own changing body. It is almost as if they fear a sex change is happening to themselves, without their permission, overnight. They need serious, factual answers about an *adult's* choice to have a sex change. Reassure them that they cannot awake one day with a sex change and that doctors would not do a sex change on a child.

If they are intensely curious about exactly how the sex change is achieved, I

Can you be a half boy and half girl because of your hormones?

refer them to autobiographies of people who have had it done.

You may wish to point out that although the newly created person will now live their life as a male or female, they cannot reproduce. We cannot transplant the reproductive organs – ovaries, uteri, or testicles. The media fascination with the Bobbitt story has convinced many children that transplants are possible, for everything!

One recent book that tells about sex changes is *Feelings: A transsexual's explanation of a baffling condition*, by Stephanie Castle (Perceptions Press).

Cross-dressing has been explored many times on the talk shows and in music videos. Children need help to understand that these folks, transvestites and men who dress in drag (flamboyant female clothes), may not be homosexual or transgendered by medical definition. These men or women may simply enjoy dressing in the clothes of the opposite sex, or they may do it to seek attention, or as part of an act. Their orientation is often heterosexual. They do not want to be the opposite sex; they simply enjoy wearing the clothing and makeup of the opposite sex.

Several children and teens have told me that they have seen transvestites on the street, at the beach, in the park, or that they have sat next to one at a ball game. They are often relieved to hear that these folks are not dangerous and that it would not be polite to ridicule them or abuse them. Sometimes I think that what children and teens anticipate and fear is peer pressure to laugh at, mock, or even attack someone who is different. The tragedy for them is that they don't have the science or health information they need to resist that pressure and to be active agents for change in peer behavior.

No one wants their young person to be charged with harassment or assault and no one wants their child to be harassed or assaulted. Education keeps us all safe.

What Are Sex Toys?

Schools today have done a marvelous job of teaching children to read and they read everything – even the ads in the back of magazines. "Send only $19.95 for our vibrator. Choose your color. They glow in the dark!" and on, and on.

Again, honesty is the best policy. Here's what I would say:

"Some people enjoy using sex toys alone, or with a partner. A dildo is made of plastic or rubber and is usually shaped a bit like an erect penis. If it has a battery in it to make it vibrate, it is called a vibrator. Legally, they can only be sold to adults, not to children.

You might like to remind your child that when he or she is an adult, they may choose to use sex toys, or not. The health information to keep in mind is that the toys must be clean. Some viruses, especially hepatitis, can survive for long periods of time on the toys and are capable of infecting or reinfecting the user. HIV, the virus that is associated with AIDS, is fragile and cannot survive outside the body when exposed to air.

What's a vibrator?
What's a Dil Doe?

Some people enjoy the toys and others do not. It is a personal choice.

What Are Bust Enlargers?
What Is a Penis Stretcher?
Do They Work?

Ads for these devices are often found in magazines and newspapers. Children can read and they do.

Devices, creams, lotions, diets, exercises, and pills do not work to enlarge anyone's breasts or penis. They only work

Are penis pumpers healty, and do they work?

to enlarge the seller's bank account. Don't hesitate to laugh with your child about the silliness of all the fantasy surrounding big breasts and giant penises.

I remember reading somewhere that out of every 100 breast surgeries done in the United States, 70 were done as reductions, only 30 for augmentation. Big breasts can give a woman a lot of physical pain and discomfort.

And you know the line about penis size, don't you? It is not the size of the wand, it is the magic in it that counts!

PART THREE

Helping Your Children Stay Healthy

9

The Sexually Active Teen

How does sex complicate relationships?

How do we know when we are ready to have sex?

How do you feel meg, about Abortions?
← Should the be a loud

Do you have to have sex with someone to show that you like them?

When are you ready for sex? This is probably one of the most common questions I hear from older teens, and it is one that adults should be asking themselves much more often than they do.

Naturally, age is important, for legal reasons. There *are* laws you know! So first, *both* people must be of legal age.

But age is also important because young bodies and minds may not be ready. Boys may not have an adult-size penis and, as a result, a condom may not fit properly. Or they may be too young to maintain an erection long enough. This physical immaturity can mean that the condom doesn't stay on properly and that the act of intercourse is a frustrating disappointment. Sadly, for many adults, their bad experiences in adolescent years get repeated over and over again in adulthood.

Then there's the emotional aspect of sexual relationships. Emotionally, in today's world, teens – and many adults – are not ready for sex, the most intimate human relationship. We may have all kinds of contraceptives to prevent pregnancy and STDs, but we don't have a pill to prevent emotional hurt. People can carry the scars and hurts like wounds that fester and sabotage all future relationships.

How do you know when you are ready to have sex and what if you aren't and your partner is.

Are You Ready for Sex?

Before you ask that question, you need to know whether or not the relationship is a mature and healthy one. How do you know that? By talking and asking questions. Below, I have listed some of the questions that teens and adults might ask themselves and, more importantly, their partners. Teens often say, "I could never sit down and ask my boy/girl friend these questions, I'd be way too embarrassed."

I respond, "Then you are not ready to have sex, and that is a good thing to know about yourself! It is not good enough to sit in the privacy of your bedroom and ask yourself these questions. Even if all of your answers indicate that you are ready for a sexual relationship, you are only one person in the equation. There is at least one other person, your partner, plus all the other people with whom you live and work."

Here, then, on the next page, are the questions.

What if the guy doesn't want to wear a condom but you want him to?

IF YOU LIKE SOMEONE DOES IT MEAN IF THEY LIKE YOU, YOU HAVE TO HAVE SEX WITH THEM?

Are You Ready to Have Sex?

1. How long have you been friends? Is it long enough to know that you are compatible? Do you have many shared values and goals?

2. Has there been any force, violence, name calling, humiliation, controlling, manipulation, guilt, or shame used against you in this relationship? If there has been, *end the relationship now!*

3. Can you have fun together without having sex?

4. Can you truly be yourself or do you have to put on an act? Can you be honest about yourself and still feel comfortable and safe? What about your partner?

5. Are you hiding anything about yourself, your family, your job, your finances, your past relationships?

6. Are you proud of this friendship? Have you each met the other's family and friends? You don't have to like them all, but it is not a good sign if you *dislike* them all.

7. Will you be embarrassed, mortified, if anyone finds out that you're having sex? If you can't be proud of yourself, *don't do it!*

8. Are you being pressured, by yourself, to prove something? Are you being pressured by your partner? Are you being pressured by your friends, or by society?

9. Are you trying to keep the relationship? Would you stay together if you didn't have sex, or couldn't have sex?

10. Are you both able to take responsibility for contraception and protection against STDs? That means using a condom, as well (perhaps) as using another contraceptive. Who is paying for the protection? You must use it every single time – can you agree?

11. Are you both willing and able to go to the doctor for check-ups and tests? Can you both afford medical care and prescriptions, if necessary? Could you tell your partner honestly, without blame, if you were infected? When in doubt, *abstain!*

12. Are you both prepared for an unplanned pregnancy? Are you certain that your values, as a couple, are compatible?

For Parents with a Sexually Active Teen

What can you do if you have a teen who is sexually active and you feel powerless to end the activity?

I expect that your first concern will be that your teen, and his or her partner, are as safe as possible from physical harm.

Here are some questions you should be asking yourself as a parent.

First, are they using a condom? It is not good enough to have the girl on the pill. Impress upon them the danger of STDs and that when you have sex with one person, you are having sex with all their previous partners, plus *their* partners! Teens often swear that they were virgins at the start of a relationship, or that they are now mutually monogamous. They may "forget" previous partners, incidents of abuse, or chronic but silent infections such as hepatitis. They may have sexually immature doctors who don't give them factual information about infections. One 15-year-old told me that when she asked her doctor how she got chlamydia the doctor said, "Oh, everybody has it these days; it's in the air."

Second, are they prepared for an unplanned pregnancy? Many teens do not understand how easy it is to get pregnant. There are no guaranteed safe days. It is possible to become pregnant *anytime*, especially when periods are not regular (monthly). Most women ovulate (release the ovum/egg) 14–16 days before the beginning of their next period. Most girls, when their periods are getting established, or when they are under stress, or dieting, or exercising heavily, or taking other medications, cannot predict when their next period will come.

The pill does not protect perfectly. Because of their busy lives, girls do not

Can a girl get pregnant while having her period?

If your on the pill and you get pregnant is this dangerous for the baby?

always take the pill at the same time every day. They don't always get a thorough explanation about taking the pill either. Several over-the-counter medicines and some prescribed medications can interfere with the effectiveness of the pill. These include antacids, analgesics, antibiotics, antihistamines, and even alcohol. If the girl is on the pill and doesn't realize she's become pregnant, and therefore continues to take the pill, it does not seem to harm the baby, especially in the beginning of the pregnancy.

About Abortions

Some parents take me by surprise with their own casual comments, such as, "Well, she can get an abortion." When it actually comes down to it, the parent may suddenly be confronted with the thought, "Oh my, this is my grandchild." I think that many people are not prepared for the deep emotions that can arise around the issue of abortion.

I like to impress upon boys that they are not wearing the condom for the girl, but to protect themselves. Who wants to be a father? Some shrug off the fatherhood question saying, "Oh, she can get an abortion."

hi I'm 16 now I just turned 16. In 3 months I would of been a mom but I had an abortion. I feel I didn't do the right thing. did I?

This is a great opportunity to do some serious talking. First, abortions may not be easily available. Who, legally, is going to give consent? Your mother? Who is going to pay for it? Ask your son if he understands the emotional impact on the girl and on himself.

In law, in most jurisdictions, the woman decides what to do about an unwanted or unplanned pregnancy. Many teenage boys have never thought about this. When I bring it up, they are outraged. "Hey, Meg, no fair. What if Joe's girl decides to have an abortion? Then he is off the hook. If my girlfriend decides to keep the baby, you mean I have to support the kid until it's 19? How come I don't have a say?" One teenage boy said, "Why does the guy have to pay money? Just stick the kid in an orphanage!"

My reply is, "It is your penis and your sperm. You are in charge of where they go. If you don't want to be a father, don't have sex." One ten-year-old girl asked a powerful question in her fifth grade class. "I don't understand about condoms. If you don't want a baby, why don't you keep your sperm to yourself?"

Of course, the teenage boy or man can sometimes be shattered when his girlfriend decides to have an abortion and he wants to keep the baby. Some rather amazing contradictions arise. Here is a typical conversation.

"If my girlfriend doesn't want the baby, I will take it."

"Who will look after it for you, since you say you want to graduate?"

"Oh, my mom will help me."

"Does your mom work?"

"Yes."

"Is she happy about the baby?"

"Well, she doesn't know yet and she's going to kill me when she finds out."

I like to suggest that they might *ask* their mothers if they'd quit work to look after this baby well before they begin to think about starting a pregnancy.

Let's be fair. It is not all doom and gloom. Some families pull together and everybody, including the baby, turns out fine. But every teen parent I have ever met says that if they could do it over again, they would not have had sex at all, let alone a baby.

Also, some teens deliberately set out to become mothers or fathers. There are a million reasons for having sex and hundreds more for getting pregnant. What we all hope for is informed choices and health for all. It seems to be that education is the key.

One last thing. It is possible for a teen, or a woman, to continue menstruating through her pregnancy. These menstrual periods are not usually normal; they usually have a lighter flow and are associated with other signs and symptoms of pregnancy (nausea, fatigue, sore breasts, etc.). Pregnancy kits from the store can help you sort out whether or not you are pregnant. They will not read positive until two weeks after conception (sperm meets ovum). If there is any doubt, see a doctor.

10

Sexually Transmitted Diseases (STDs)

how many people can you safely have sex with?

Does pot and steroos shrink your testicals

How does aids kill you

How does it get transfered

My Dad always scrotches his testicles Dose that meen he has herpes

Sexually transmitted diseases have become much better known and understood by the medical community in the last few decades. For most of human history, we only knew about syphilis and gonorrhea and we called those two VD, or venereal diseases. After the Second World War, when antibiotics became available, both were curable and also reportable. That meant that doctors who treated patients for VD had to report those treatments to public health officials. Names of sexual contacts were supplied too. In my early nursing career, I worked with older public health nurses who had experience being sent to an address to tell the person that their name had been given as a sexual partner of an infected person and that they should seek treatment for themselves.

Gradually through the 1960s, '70s, and '80s, more and more organisms, bacteria, and viruses were recognized. It soon became evident that many of these were transmitted by sexual contact; not by toilet seats, door knobs, drinking fountains, or by holding hands.

When I am teaching students, I point out to them that there are now more than 50 STDs, and that eight of them are potentially fatal. It is always fun and interesting to brainstorm that list of "The Big Eight" with them. Ready? Here they are: HIV/AIDS, hepatitis B and C, genital warts or HPV (human papilloma virus), chlamydia, herpes, gonorrhea, and syphilis. I have smiled quietly to myself as students offer other diseases, such as "herbies," cramps, head lice, and hemorrhoids – none of which are fatal!

Let's take "The Big Eight" one by one.

HIV/AIDS

If you become HIV positive, meaning that you have contracted the virus but are not yet ill, you are still able to give the virus to any sexual partner. It is important to impress upon any age child or teen that you can only get HIV by having sexual intercourse with an HIV-positive partner, or by infected blood, usually from sharing HIV contaminated or "dirty" needles with an infected person.

Too many people believe that multiple partners causes AIDS. You could (if you were sexually immature or uneducated) have sex with 1,000 people and, if none of them had HIV, you wouldn't get AIDS. Sometimes young children think that any one act of sexual intercourse will give you AIDS. Too many teens believe that only gay men can get HIV. Believe me, it's sad when I meet a heterosexual teen or woman who says, "Sure we did anal sex (to avoid a pregnancy), but we're not gay, I can't be HIV positive." We are still hearing such things, even in these so-called "enlightened times."

I sit on an advisory board to a women-and-AIDS project. The staff tell us about daily phone calls from teens and women requesting anonymous testing. They say they have asked the family doctor or gynecologist and the doctor has replied, "You, Mrs. Jones? Why do you need an AIDS test? You're not sleeping around are you? You've been married for five years; you don't need to be tested."

Of course, the teen or woman is not going to tell her story at that point. She may have just heard that a previous partner has tested positive; she may have found out that her husband has had an affair; she may have had one herself. Doctors are not always sexually mature themselves and I have had them say to me, "I don't have to test any of my patients. They are all professionals."

Sharing contaminated needles for IV drugs is not common among teens in every

If some one bleeds on you and they don't have aids will you get aids

Couldn't you get aids by kissing someone

community, but another pattern of teen behavior *is* being seen more often in every community: I'm talking about needle sharing to inject steroids. It is usually boys who buy the drugs and needles, in or around gyms. Too often, they share them with girls.

First, let's look at why teens, and sometimes even younger children, take steroids. For boys, the attraction is the belief that you will get bigger muscles, a more sexually attractive body. For the girls, the belief is that steroids will make you slim and therefore more attractive. When they tell me this, often in a class full of others, without any sense of shame or guilt, I love to say them, "Why would anyone take such risks to make their body sexually attractive and then not have any equipment to work with?" They need to know that steroids can adversely affect sexual organs and increase aggression. On top of all that, I remind them that they could get HIV. "Then how sexually attractive are you going to be?"

Tattooing (body art) also poses a risk, especially of hepatitis, if contaminated needles are shared.

Can steroids shrink your testicles?

It may sound extreme, but there are days when I believe that the advertising world – with its constant preoccupation with body shape and size, its sexualization of children, its unrealistic and false images of human bodies, and its constant use of sex to sell everything from toothpaste to chain saws – is killing our children. We need more sexually mature adults to call a halt.

Some children and teens think that if you get AIDS, or any other STD, you can get rid of it by having sex with someone else and passing it on like a parcel. It should go without saying, and yet it must be said:

"This is not true." The virus is living throughout your *whole* body; you cannot get rid of it by having sex.

Hepatitis B and C

Hepatitis is now nicknamed the "alphabet disease" because the virus keeps mutating and, with new technology, doctors can identify more virus strains. Viruses that infect the liver are called hepatitis. Some of them, such as hepatitis A, are very infectious and can easily be transmitted by saliva, for example. Hepatitis B and C are now known to be mainly transmitted by sexual intercourse. They can be fatal in their acute stage, but most people can overcome the virus and be well again. Some people become chronic carriers, and although they are well, they can pass the virus to sexual partners. There are vaccines now for several types of hepatitis.

The virus can also kill if it causes liver cancer. Some possible symptoms are fatigue, nausea, jaundice, and pain.

Never hesitate to consult your doctor whenever you have doubts about your own health or a partner's health.

Genital Warts

Genital warts are caused by HPV (human papilloma virus). The virus is passed from an infected partner to another partner through intimate sexual activity. It may take months, even years, before a wart appears. Many people don't know they've ever been exposed because the wart may be inside the vagina, on the cervix, under the foreskin, or so small that you can hardly see it. The warts can be treated by a doctor, without pain, while they are small. Left untreated they may need to be removed surgically. Left untreated they also increase the risk of cancers of the reproductive organs. Apart from smoking, HPV is also the leading cause of mouth and throat cancer. This is very worrying when we see teens using oral sex as a way to avoid pregnancy.

I always tell teens that genital warts is my favorite, potentially fatal STD because of the cancer risk. They are convinced that this is proof that I am a pervert. "Gross, Meg, you have a favorite fatal STD!"

It is only my favorite STD because I know exactly what teens are going to say when I write genital warts on the blackboard. "Oh yeah, Meg. How can genital warts be catching? Who would ever have sex with a guy who has warts all over his penis?"

Probably no one! But that is not where the warts grow in the beginning. They commonly grow under the foreskin – if he does not pull the foreskin back and look at his penis when he is washing, he may not know that they are there. They are tiny and painless. In females, the warts can be up high inside the vagina and, if she is not honest with her doctor about her sexual activity, the doctor may not test for them. Most often, they are first seen or felt at the opening of the vagina. Be sure to self-check by feeling and looking.

Are private part warts can taj us

It's important for all sexually active women to have regular pap smears in order to find any changes in the cervix that could potentially lead to a cancer. If diagnosed early, it's easily treatable.

Unfortunately, once you have HPV it may be in your body for life. Recurring warts can be treated, but you will always be in danger of infecting a partner.

Gonorrhea and Chlamydia

Gonorrhea and chlamydia are commonly called "the silent diseases" because the majority of people who are infected will not have symptoms. Guys are lucky in a biological way; they urinate and have sex with their penis, so the infections can cause burning when they urinate. In fact, a urinalysis can often diagnose the infections in males. Why can't a urinalysis always detect the infections in women? I love asking children, teens, and adults that question. Everyone looks back at me with blank stares. "Because we don't pee out of our vaginas!" Immediately, a few in the class or audience will relax, laugh, sit back and say "Of course, how could I have forgotten that?" But still, the majority of each group looks even more tense, puzzled, and says, "They (we) don't?"

Many, many people are still confused by the saying, "Boys have a penis, girls have a vagina." Females do not urinate out of their vaginas; the urine comes out of the urethra, the opening at the front of the genitals, not out of the vagina, which is in the middle. Babies come out of vaginas!

Gonorrhea and chlamydia, left untreated in males, can climb the penis, infect the prostate gland (where semen is made), and eventually descend to the testicles causing infertility. Rarely are they ever fatal for men. They can, however, cause fatalities in females.

In females, the organisms can proceed from the vagina, through the uterus (remember the tiny size of these parts), through the fallopian tubes, and out into the abdomen. When this happens it is called PID or pelvic inflammatory disease. Doctors have nicknamed it "pus in dere."

Let me pause here to remind you of the films or slides you may have seen at school on menstruation. Do you remember that the uterus filled the screen? The tubes were as big as garden hoses! In fact, the tubes are about as big as the lead in a pencil. Sperm are microscopic, so they go through easily.

If chlamydia or gonorrhea have infected the fallopian tubes and left scars, it may still be possible for the sperm to go through and fertilize an ovum. The fertilized ovum, however, is so much bigger that it may get stuck in the tube. As the ovum grows larger, it can rupture the tube and cause massive bleeding. Each year, over 1,000 women in North America die from tubal or ectopic pregnancies; this is to say nothing of the many more thousands who survive, but who may be left infertile or chronically ill.

Too often, the infection has no symptoms. It is possible for males and females to walk around for years with these infections without knowing it. All the while, they may be infecting other sexual partners. The scars (called lesions) in the abdomen can cause serious problems later in her life.

A sexually active teen or adult needs to be honest with their doctor about sexual activity and ask to be tested with each new partner. Sometimes people say, "But I am in love with this person, we're only sleeping with each other." I know that it is almost a cliché, but when you have sex with one person, you are exposing yourself to all the other diseases that their previous partners may have had, and their partners, and their partners. Girls don't always tell guys that they are not virgins. They say that a previous act of intercourse doesn't count. We were not in love; we only did it once; I didn't have an orgasm; on and on! I have even had teenage boys and young men say, "Well that one didn't count 'cuz she was ugly, or fat, or everybody slept with her...so that doesn't count!"

Can a person have a disease but not know it for the rest of their lives?

There are occasional cases of resistant gonorrhea, but generally, all gonorrhea and chlamydia infections can be cured in the early stages with antibiotics. If you have any questions, talk to your doctor or go to a medical clinic or an STD clinic. Service is confidential and *you* get to tell your partner. No public health official goes out to knock on doors with STD reports anymore.

I remember a 15-year-old girl who burst out in class one day when I was putting the list of STDs on the board.

"Hey, I've had that and it's not fair. I've been taking antibiotics all month because I got it twice this month. I didn't know that chlamydia was an STD." She went on to tell us all that this was her first boyfriend, "So how come I got chlamydia twice?"

I asked if she had told her boyfriend about the infection the first time.

"Oh, no," she explained. "I didn't want him to think I might have given him a disease."

Several other students now spoke up. "If you were a virgin, then he gave it to you," they said.

"Oh, yeah, he did!" she exclaimed.

"Well, you went back and had sex with him again and he gave it back to you."

"Oh yeah," she said again.

At this point, I asked, "Didn't your doctor tell you to tell your boyfriend and that he should be treated too?"

Now she got angry. "No, he didn't. I had never heard of chlamydia before and I asked him what it was and he said everybody had it these days."

Biting back my thoughts about her doctor, I said, "Well, will you tell your boyfriend now that you're on your second batch of antibiotics."

"Oh, no, I don't have to," she said with a happy grin. "I've broken up with him."

"But," I spluttered, "then he's out there giving chlamydia to all the other girls he's having sex with."

"Oh, yeah," she said, thinking slowly.

At this point, all the others in the class began to call to her. "Who is it? Want me to tell him for you?" "Yeah, who is it, what's his name?" Some even began suggesting names.

I hope that this very personal disclosure brought the seriousness of infection home to them all.

Symptoms, if there *are* any, may include burning when you urinate, or a puslike discharge from the penis or the vagina. Sometimes there is pain during sex. But rather than sit at home and wonder about symptoms, go to your doctor and get tested. Don't take chances.

And don't rush to assume that your present partner has been unfaithful if you *do* test positive. He or she may have contracted it years before they met you, or you could have been carrying it yourself from a previous partner. The most important thing is treatment!

Genital Herpes

The genital herpes virus is similar to the herpes virus that causes the common cold sore on the lips. Sometimes these viruses change places when people have oral sex.

The herpes virus can lie dormant in your body for years. The majority of people who have an outbreak of herpes only have it once. There is a prescription medicine that can be very helpful in decreasing the pain from the blisterlike lesions. The sores may not be visible outside the body, so it is always prudent to be honest with your partner and doctor about a previous infection.

What is Herpes?

If a baby is born through the vagina when the mother is having a genital herpes outbreak, that baby may get very sick. A Cesarean section may be performed by the doctor to avoid this possibility.

Persons with a genital herpes outbreak rarely die, but, once in a long while, the virus can migrate to other vital areas of the body and occasionally *that* can be fatal.

The herpes virus has been thought to increase the risk of cervical cancer. Today, STD experts are warning that any sexually transmitted infection increases the risk of contracting HIV and other life-threatening conditions.

There are herpes hotlines to call for further information, and many of the larger cities and university centers have herpes clinics. Do not hesitate to seek expert advice; it is usually free.

Syphilis

Syphilis is probably the least common STD, but the World Health Organization has noted an alarming increase around the world, particularly in Southeast Asia. In many countries, it is commonly associated with HIV.

Syphilis can usually be cured with antibiotics, but of course, testing must be done to establish its presence.

If syphilis is not treated, it can migrate throughout the body, from the original genital sores, and cause insanity and death years later. Again, take every genital problem, even a small sore, to the doctor. Get tested, tell your partner, take the medicine, and save lives!

Summary

This chapter is not meant to be a medical text on sexually transmitted diseases. It is simply meant to raise your awareness. Please, go to your doctor, a medical clinic, or an STD clinic if you have any questions about your health. Testing can be anonymous, even for teens. Treatment is usually simple, and full confidence will be yours.

Resources

Don't rely on books and magazine articles for accurate information, especially if they are more than six to 12 months old. The best resource is a medical school, its library, your local STD clinic.

11

What Happens in the Doctor's Office

Can a doctor tell if you masturbate or if you have had digital sex?

Do you have to go to the gyno before you're sexually active?

Why do women bleed the first time?

Is it true when you wear tampons you break your virgina openings?

Most of us, even though we may consider ourselves to be mature, find going to the doctor pretty intimidating. This is especially true if we're going for a sexual health exam. How can we help our teens?

First, we can tell them what to expect. Fear of the unknown plays a major role in keeping teens, and many adults, out of the doctor's office. I have provided a description of a typical examination, for both males and females, below. Please share this information with your teen.

Second, for girls, if it is possible and if they'd prefer it, try to find them a female doctor. But I also need to add a word of caution about this. I've met a few female doctors who were horrible and many male doctors who were fantastic. Gender doesn't always matter, but if that is what it takes to get her (or him) to the doctor, do what you can to help.

Teens don't always want to go to the same family doctor as their parents, so try to be understanding about this. Promise them confidentiality if that is what it takes and be sure to tell the doctor.

Finally, don't forget to hold up your own shining example. Parents who go to the doctor without complaining whenever it is necessary do a great job of modeling responsible behavior. *Everyone* has to go at one time or another, so *go!*

Males

Most males, in my experience, are reluctant to visit a doctor. They tell me that they are scared, that they don't know what to expect, and that they are really frightened that they will suffer embarrassment and pain.

Doctors have not been very good at calming these fears and have often rushed through the exams in order to lessen the agony. Of course, guys occasionally share the agony with their buddies and then rumors, stories, guilt, and shame are passed along, person to person, generation to generation.

Let's talk about what happens and why. Here's how I would describe an examination for a teen.

First, the doctor should take a medical history. That means you just talk. The doctor will probably ask you the following questions: Are you healthy? Do you have any general health problems? Are you sexually active? How often do you have sex (usually meaning sexual intercourse)? Do you have sex with one, or more than one partner? What kind of sex do you have, and what kind of protection do you use? What protection does your partner use? Is your sexual experience satisfactory? And finally, do you have any pain or worries at the moment?

What if a doctor asked to see your private spots. Is that okay?

Doctors, by the way, should not assume that you are heterosexual or exclusively gay. Be prepared for the question and be prepared to be honest.

Next, the doctor must look at and examine your genitals, so you have to take your pants off. You should be given a gown or an examining drape to cover yourself. The doctor may cup your scrotum in his or her hand, feel your testicles, and ask you to cough. They do this to check the health of your testicles. Do they move when you cough? Are they smooth? Are there any lumps, bruises, warts, sores, or swellings? The doctor will review the testicular self-exam. All males should check their own testicles at least monthly.

The doctor will look at the penis for any similar problems and to see if there is any abnormal discharge. The doctor must check under the foreskin for scars, sores, and warts.

Once that area has been checked, the doctor may do a rectal examination. To do this, he or she will have you lie down on the examining table. Don't panic, breathe deeply, try to stay relaxed. The doctor will put on a latex rubber glove, lubricate it with some gel, and then put one finger in your anus and rectum. This is done to examine the prostate gland for signs of infection, enlargement, or lumps. It only takes a few seconds. Your penis might become erect. This is normal. It does not mean that you or the doctor are perverts. A good doctor would explain all this to you before the exam starts, or talk to you continuously throughout the examination. Some don't, so it is your responsibility to be sexually mature and to be informed.

If there is any indication of infection, the doctor will ask you for a urine and/or stool sample. He or she may also swab your anus and your throat. You must be honest with the doctor (even if the doctor does not ask) about which sexual activities you have had: vaginal, anal, and/or oral sex. Remember that the STDs can grow anywhere that there is sexual contact or exchange of body fluids. And of course, admit to any needle sharing.

When should you go to a doctor to check the prostate gland

Doctors are not in business to be judgmental. If you think that your doctor is judging you, change doctors!

Your doctor may also do an abdominal exam, checking your liver and spleen in particular for signs of infection. Blood tests may be ordered.

A thorough checkup for STDs takes an average of 15 minutes. It can save your life and the life of your partner. Drag yourself into sexual maturity and go!

If you have never had sex and are healthy in all other respects, you should probably have the above exam done when you reach 18–20 years of age. All being well, you may not need to be examined again until you become sexually active. Then, you will need to be examined again with each new sexual partner, or if you learn that your partner is not monogamous.

A very good book for males about sexual health is *Private Parts: An Owner's Guide*, by Dr. Y. Taguchi (McClelland & Stewart).

Females

This is how I would describe the need for a physical examination, and the examination itself, to a teenage girl.

If you are healthy and a virgin, you do not need to have a gynecological exam until you are 19 or 20 years old, and then not again until you begin having sexual intercourse. A pelvic exam is necessary to check your ovaries and the uterus. A pap smear (samples of cells taken from the cervix, the opening to the uterus) is necessary once you have had intercourse. Once you are sexually active, you should be examined with each new sexual partner. If you are certain that your relationship is mutually monogamous, you should still be examined annually. Guys are lucky – most of their genitalia is on the outside and easy to examine. Your genitals are inside the abdomen and so the examinations are more invasive.

When should you start seeing a gynacologist?

First, as with males, the doctor should take a medical history. That means you just talk. The doctor will probably ask you the same questions he or she asks of boys: Are you healthy? Do you have any general health problems? Are you sexually active? How often do you have sex? Do you have sex with one, or more than one partner? What kind of sex do you have, and what kind of protection do you use? What protection does your partner use? Is your sexual experience satisfactory? Do you have an orgasm? And finally, do you have any pain or worries at the moment?

As in examinations for males, the doctor should not assume that you are heterosexual or exclusively lesbian. Be prepared for the question and be prepared to be honest.

Next, the doctor will probably leave you so you can get undressed. When he or she comes back into the room, you will be asked to lie on your back on the examining table and to put your heels up, next to your buttocks. Personally, I would ask not to put my legs up in stirrups. They are not necessary and I'd feel too trapped. However, if your doctor uses them and you don't mind, it is your decision – *not the doctor's!* It certainly doesn't hurt to ask the doctor if he or she could do the examination without using the stirrups.

The doctor may use a plastic disposable instrument called a speculum, to enable him or her to see inside your vagina. Some doctors use a metal one that is sterilized after each patient. If a metal speculum is used, the doctor should warm it under the hot water tap before inserting it. You do not have to accept a freezing cold speculum inserted into your vagina!

Let me pause here for a word about the hymen. Some, perhaps many, baby girls are born without a hymen. Most hymens get torn and stretched painlessly and without bleeding as a little girl grows. No one, including a doctor, can say with absolute certainty whether a girl or woman has or has not had sexual intercourse.

Of course, if sperm or semen are present in or around the vagina, if there are STD organisms present, or, if in the case of sexual assault, bruises, tearing or bleeding are evident, those things indicate that the woman or girl is not a virgin. Pregnancy may occur without penetration and is not an indicator.

The old myths about hymens have caused much misery in our societies, particularly for girls and women. The old crudity about "popping cherries" has to go. That ugliness is much more about ignorance of female anatomy than about virginity. Only the male or the female themselves can say if they are virgins. And why would anyone, other than your doctor, want to know anyway?

Returning to the examination, once the doctor has inserted the speculum, he or she will look at your vagina. It should look pink, moist, and healthy, just like the inside of your mouth – only more wrinkled. Then the doctor will take a wooden stick (a bit like a tongue depressor) and scrape a few cells off your cervix, the "mouth" of the uterus. Those cells get wiped onto a glass slide and are sent to a cytology lab where they are tested for cancer or pre-cancerous cells. This procedure is called a pap smear. It does not test for STDs.

is it true that you won't bleed after your first time having sex if you're over 16?

Second, the doctor will swab the vagina with two cotton swabs. The swabs go to a different lab to check for STD organisms. Be sure to tell the doctor if you've had digital, anal, or oral sex, so that these extra swabs can be done.

After removing the speculum, the doctor will then put on a latex rubber glove and insert two fingers into your vagina; the doctor's other hand goes on your abdomen. This procedure is called the pelvic exam and the doctor is checking for abnormalities in the uterus and ovaries. These exams are not painful, but not always comfortable either. They take less than a minute or two and could save your life.

How old are you when you have a pap shmere? What happens during one?

You may be asked for urine and blood samples as well, but remember, a urine sample is not a good indicator of STDs because the urine does not come out of the vagina.

While you are there, the doctor should also check for breast lumps and will review the breast self-examination that girls and women should do at least monthly.

Don't be afraid or too embarrassed to ask questions, to ask for explanations, and to ask for a nurse, a friend, or your partner to be present with you during the examination. You are entitled to choices and to a full understanding of why certain questions may be asked of you, and why specific procedures must be done. Doctors usually like it when teens care and know enough to ask them questions.

The whole examination usually takes 15 to 30 minutes, but you can always ask for more time. If you have many questions, the doctor may book another appointment.

How long does a doctors check up take!

We all need to be sexually mature in the doctor's office because the doctor may *not* be! Take charge – it's your money and your life.

Good books are available to help you learn about female sexual health, pap smears, and other examinations. I particularly recommend *A New View of a Woman's Body*, by the Federation of Feminist Women's Health Centers (Feminist Health Press).

PART
FOUR

Communicating
Your
Values

12

Family Values

Do you think that your job is just taking away the job of our parents telling us about love and sex? since we trust and look up to them.

When should Dating Start

The joy and challenge of raising children will encourage you to clarify your family values, sometimes with the speed of lightning.

In many of my parent audiences, parents have raised their hands and asked, "What do I say?" Several times when I have asked the parent, "What are your values?" they have replied, "I don't know." "What if my values are not like everyone else's?" "How do I say what my values are?"

Some parents have told me that they were perfectly happy with the values they were raised with in the 1970s, until they had children in the 1980s or 1990s and suddenly those 1970s values no longer seemed appropriate. Changing or adapting older values can seem like a betrayal of parents or institutions that nurtured us.

Perhaps asking ourselves some questions can help: questions such as "Is this a nurturing value or could it be hurtful, even dangerous to someone?"

For instance, what can you say when television shows or movies condone or even promote teenage sexual activity and pregnancy? Many parents have said, "I hate it when that turns up in shows that I am watching with my kids, but do I say something?" If you say nothing, change the channel, or put your hand over the child's eyes, the child is confused too. Children tell me that they think it might be okay "because my parents never say anything," or the children report being completely puzzled: "Why don't they talk to me?"

I suggest that parents ask themselves, "What message do I want to give my child?" One mom talked about her 15-year-old niece who was pregnant. "How can I help my children, who adore this girl, understand that teen parenting is not a good idea?"

I asked her if she wanted her own children to be teen parents.

"Of course not."

"Then you're going to have to say that your niece is not a good role model."

As cute as a new baby is, as much fun as baby showers are, there is a price to pay in this situation. What about school; shelter for mom and babe? Where is the father? Who will care for the baby?... The young adoring cousins don't have to condemn their teenage cousin, but they can understand that having sex and babies at 15 is not a great idea.

Another parent called me and said, "I have just discovered that my 20-year-old son is having sex with his girlfriend, in his bedroom, in our house. How can I get him to stop?"

My first question was, "Did you ever tell him that your family values include no sexual activity until you are independent?"

"Well no," she said. "We didn't ever say that to him and he's told us that we never said that."

This man and his wife have several options, of course. They can say *now*, "These are the house rules." Since they pay the mortgage and stock the fridge, their rules and values come first. They also need to have some serious discussions with their son and perhaps with his girlfriend. Why are these values important to this family? What are the parents worried about? What options does the son have?

I'd like to suggest to every family that they start talking about family values at the preschool age, and that if, for example, your family value is "sex belongs in marriage," then you must say that 500 times between the age of three and 30!

An old adage says, "If children are not taught or encouraged to believe in something, they will believe in anything."

A story from my colleague, Alice Bell, speaking to a primary class:

Alice: Sex is only for grownups and some families believe that you only have sex when you marry. You children need to know what the rules are for your family.

Child (shouting): NO FEET ON THE COUCH!

Dating

Parents tell me that they are shocked at how young dating begins. Children tell me that they feel pressured into dating long before they are ready.

Families who talk about dating in the primary grades can support their children's resistance to peer pressure. Even joking about it can be helpful: "When you go out on your first date, when you are 25, Daddy and I will come too, okay?"

What is the appropriate dating age within your values? Will you encourage group dates first, parents driving? Will you want to meet or know the date's parents? Does the boy have to come to the door to collect your daughter? Will there be rules about where they go, when your child must come home, who pays?

The best time to begin to clarify your values and to talk with your children is before these issues arrive. It is never too early and television and movies provide many opportunities to talk.

what is the proper age to start dateing

You might want to consider a house rule that there will be no entertaining friends in bedrooms. Parents don't visit with their friends in their bedrooms, why would you allow your children or teens to do that? University students have told me about instances of making out in their bedrooms, when things got out of control and assaults and rapes happened. The victim was afraid to call for help for fear that the parent would make a scene and embarrass them. I know that the teens will say that they want privacy from their younger sibling, but parents need to ask, "Privacy for what?"

Television

What are your family values when it comes to television? Is it on all the time? Do you limit the hours or the shows? Do you ever question the content? Who controls the remote control? Are you conscious of your own reactions and behaviors while watching television with your children? Do you swear at referees, make sexist, racist, or homophobic remarks about people appearing on shows? Which "good guys" do you cheer for, and who are the "bad guys"?

Children often need adults to help them appreciate and discriminate moral and ethical behavior, not only among those they see on television, but among those with whom they watch TV. Just as road rage isn't good for children as passengers in a car, adult viewing behavior can affect children even more than the questionable content they might see in shows and in ads.

Here are some questions you might want to take some time to consider: How much violence is acceptable when we watch television as a family? Do my children understand the difference between fantasy and real life?

My seven-year-old grandson Nicholas showed more maturity than many adults when he said, "People need to understand that the *Power Rangers* are a story and you're not supposed to act like that in real life." There are numerous adults who need to reflect on that wisdom when it comes to wrestling shows and violent movies – these things do *not* depict real life!

When it comes to sex on television, you need to explain that the sex is acted, that it is not real. So often, sexism, sexuality, and violence are plainly evident (or implied) and commingled, and we can be guilty of condoning that by our silence. Is that how we want our daughters to be treated? Is that how we want our sons to act?

In the T.V is its true that the men and women is doing sex?

Don't sit there in worried silence; *talk* to your children. Even if you don't know exactly what to say, talk about your uncomfortable feelings, your worries about the message that you think is being given. What is the message that you *wish* was there?

Moms and dads don't always have to agree, in my opinion. Children quickly learn in their very young years that there is a wide variety of opinion in the world. Dad may truly live for *Monday Night Football* and Mom adores *As The World Turns*, but let us hope children joining their parents on the couch are learning and observing respectful attitudes as well as critical viewing skills.

You may also want to consider using the "Off" button more. Some families don't allow any television viewing on school nights or during daylight hours on weekends. Some ban TV altogether, or ration their viewing, giving a child a choice: they can watch whatever they like after school, but only for one hour. There are many values that are there for us to choose, but perhaps the least used and understood is that of the "Off" button.

Condoms and Birth Control

"Do I buy my son condoms or get my daughter on the pill, just in case?"

What are your family values? Parents have told me that their bottom line is to make certain that their teen is safe. Some teens have told me that they appreciate knowing that their parents will help them with contraceptives while other teens have said that they were insulted and hurt that their parents would offer help.

I want to emphasize again that constant talking with your children is the best way to stress your family values. Respect for others' values is also admirable, but never

---

A father told me that during W.W. II, in his hometown in Scotland, there were a lot of American soldiers and there was lots of talk about "French letters" (condoms). He asked his mother what a French letter was and she replied, "A letter from France, ye wee daft lad!"

assume that theirs may be the same as yours.

One family told me how shocked they were to discover that their daughter's boyfriend's family had very different values, even though they all attended the same church and his father was the assistant pastor. The girl's parents expected there to be no sexual activity and the boy's parents thought that boys were free to explore and experiment. It is quite possible to have teens in church on Sunday, at youth group on Thursday, and at the sexually transmitted disease clinic on Monday.

Pornography

In the "old days," like last year, the most common story I would hear was "I found a pornographic magazine in my son's bedroom." I still hear that, but more likely it will be pornography on computers and the Web, on CD-ROMs or DVDs, on videos, and children telling each other about pornography.

What are your values about pornography?

You may want to talk with your children about the exploitation, the violence, the coercion, the drugs, alcohol, STDs, and suicides that are common in the pornography industry. It is not only the actors that are being exploited, but the viewers too. Pornographers use makeup, trick photography, airbrushing, and, more commonly now, computer enhancement and manipulation. Bodies are not "real," positions can be faked, the smiles and fun are phony, and it is grueling work.

It is important for parents to understand that child abusers often use pornography to persuade children that sexual acts are acceptable and fun. Parents should,

Are kids alowed to wacth porno movies

HOW COME SEX IS ASSOCIATED WITH VIOLENT TERMS.

therefore, be open about discussing pornography so that children will feel that it is safe to tell a parent when they have been exposed to such material.

It can happen in the most unexpected places. Parents have told me how surprised they were when pornography was shown at sleep-overs, at a relative's house, at summer camp, or at sports schools. Remember that pedophiles seek employment involving children and that most abusers began exploiting children as teenagers. We must be prepared to report any teen, male or female, who acts inappropriately with children. There were often exploited or abused themselves and need help.

Computers and the Internet

Media reports of children's exposure to Internet pornography; children being abducted or enticed to meet with chat-room friends; e-mail bullying among school children; teens posting personal nude videos or seductive photos on their Blogs (web logs) and on their cell phones; and many other exploitive situations are commonplace today.

What is a parent to do? Here are some suggestions, not only from myself out of my own experience talking with parents and students, but from professionals who deal with these situations on a daily basis. Police, social workers, even computer experts have endorsed these ideas.

Do you know how people get phornography on the computer?

1. Make sure that all computers in your home are in a well-traveled area of the house, for example, the kitchen or living room, where one can keep an eye on the screen. It is not safe to have your child or teen alone in their bedroom with their own private computer with access to the Internet.

2. Always be willing to talk with your child about unsavory images or issues that they may find. Try your best not to be angry with your child. Save your energy for reporting to those who are responsible.

3. Know the technology yourself. I am appalled at parents who have cable or satellite TV and who do not know how to block channels.

   Know how to access the "History" feature of your Internet browser so that you can check the sites your child has visited. Of course, it is an easy thing to clear your browser's "history" of visited sites and some children will figure out how to do this on their own, but that alone can provide a clue that they may be visiting sites you might not approve of. If your children have been spending time surfing the net, but the "history" is consistently empty, it may be appropriate to ask them why. Also, don't forget to watch your credit card billings for unauthorized visits and charges.

   Do you know about blocking and tracking software? Net Nanny and CyberSitter are two software programs that can filter your child's access to the Internet by blocking objectionable websites, images, and language. These programs are less effective, however, at monitoring on-line chat groups, or e-mail and instant messaging programs, such as MSN Messenger and ICQ. If this is something you want to do, there is a program called e-Blaster that will record every key stroke your child types (as well as the websites they visit) and will e-mail you a report at regular intervals.

   If all of this is new to you, there are many Internet sites set up by experts in all fields that are well worth visiting and that are truly educational and instructive. Community centers and night schools have teachers and offer short courses you can access to become more computer-literate. Children seem to be born with technology skills in their DNA now, but don't let them get ahead of you. Keep abreast of them or form a partnership with your whiz-kid so that you can protect each other. Learning, as you know, should be fun.

4. Be clear with your children about the dangers of chat rooms. As I write this, two girls from British Columbia, aged 13 and 14, have just been found in Ontario, more than halfway across the country and almost a week after they first disappeared. The two were on their way to New York City and were caught when they stopped in Ontario to meet a "friend" they had met on the Internet.

   Explain that pedophiles can easily pretend to be ten years old and a friend. Teach your children not to provide *any* personal information in a chat room. Ask yourself if there are other real-life social activities that you could help your child participate in rather than interacting on a computer: sports, volunteering, dance, etc.

5. Don't forget that you need to be concerned about your children when they are away from home, too. Even if you don't have a TV or computer in your house, or a cell phone with picture technology, other kids do have them, or have access to them. Earlier this year, national newspapers reported the case of a 20-year-old man who, surreptitiously, used a cell phone to take nude photographs of his 17-year-old girlfriend and then posted those photographs on his website. Your children need to know not only that this sort of thing can happen, but that it is highly illegal. In the case above, the young man was charged with possessing, manufacturing, and distributing child pornography, and was sentenced to six months in jail.

   Every day, police find DVDs and video tapes with unspeakable child and adult pornography and it possible that your children may encounter such things, even in supposedly safe environments. There are enough stories of so-called respectable, professional people using these materials to make anyone paranoid. The best protection is openness, awareness, and education.

Remember, too, when on vacation, that many hotels provide in-room access to pay-per-view pornographic movies, which your children might access even by accident. If you ask, most hotels will block these channels from your room, or tell you how to do it yourself.

6. Finally, monitor yourself. Do you spend a lot of time on-line, in chat rooms, surfing the net? What kind of behavior are you modeling for your child?

It seems to me that the wisest parents recognize that all sorts of immoral, deviant, and uncivil behaviors are "out there," on the Internet, and in the media. Our children are best protected by education and open discussion. Never hesitate to inform your Internet service provider (ISP) when you are offended by something that you and your child find on the Internet. Above all, teach your child and train yourself not to visit those sites. Every click earns them money. Teaching children to critically evaluate any publication or depiction for sexism, racism, bullying, or disrespect is an ongoing challenge, but our children deserve to grow up with respect and safety.

What's Your Bottom Line?

I would like to see every adult and child thriving in communities and homes where respect for themselves and others is the number one principle. Of course, there may be moments when the odd swear word slips out, where an old and hurtful stereotype reappears, and when an adult behaves in a thoughtless way. Children often accept sincere apologies with much more grace than adults do.

We all struggle with old behaviors, opinions, and language patterns which are no longer socially acceptable. Parents need to demonstrate for children that the struggle is real, but that we can move on. Hitting back and draconian punishment are not helpful.

Work at establishing solid moral values for yourselves and for your children. The whole community will benefit if we gently insist that all children act respectfully, even if it is only "in our house" or "in our car." "We do not behave like that." Many adults in today's world did not learn to be civil and to uphold moral values in their own homes, where abuse or dysfunction was the norm. They learned to be respectful and thoughtful at a neighbor's house, on a soccer team, in a classroom, or at a club they attended. Treat every child with respect and dignity, and the whole community thrives.

13

Parents and Families Who Are Faithful

Does everybody have sex?!

Is it against God or religious groups to change sex if you are religious but want to change?

When people say God created us what does it mean? Because I'm pretty sure that humans make babies.

Once, after a family session during which children and parents came together to hear my presentation, a man came up to me and said, "That was wonderful; I have never heard it presented so well and I am almost sorry that I did not allow my wife and children to come."

I had an idea that this was a man of Christian fundamentalist belief; he was head of the home and had absolute control over his family. He went on: "I want to offer you one bit of constructive criticism. Please take it in the spirit that I give it." I said I would. "I think it is wonderful that you tell the children not to worry about breast cancer when they feel those lumps behind their nipples. I remember worrying myself sick about that when I was young. But you don't need to tell them that breast cancer is an adult disease because that means that you are an evolutionist and you are denying children the knowledge of God."

"Well, I think that the congregation that I worship with each Sunday would be surprised to hear that I deny children the knowledge of God," I replied. "Could you tell me what you mean?" He was clearly surprised by my church affiliation, but he went on.

In a fourth grade class:
Child: What's a hooker?

Meg: First, who knows the scientific name?

Another child, waving her hand excitedly: I know, I know. It's a Protestant!

"Well, if you say that men can get breast cancer, then you are saying that men evolved, but that's not true. God made men perfect. Therefore, you are an evolutionist, and since evolutionists do not believe in God, you deny children the chance to know God."

What could I say? There were other parents lined up behind him waiting to talk to me and I knew that it would take a long time to get him to consider another viewpoint. So I simply shook his hand, thanked him for his honesty, and said, "You've given me something to think about."

"That's all I ask," he said warmly, and left.

Now, it would be easy to poke holes in his theory, in his theology – to dismiss him as a nut case. Three days later, however, I got a phone call from a principal of a school near the one at which I had spoken to the fundamentalist gentleman. The principal was very gracious, but he explained that, although his parent advisory council had booked me to speak at their school, he was forced to cancel the meeting.

"I'm very sorry. I know how good you are," he said. "But at church on Sunday I heard that you are an evolutionist and I cannot take a chance on that becoming an issue at 'my school.'"

I have a long waiting list, so I simply thanked him for calling and prepared to offer the dates to another school. Moments later, the parent chairperson was on the phone begging me not to cancel just yet; she was certain that the principal did not have the power to cancel the meeting that so many parents wanted. Despite their best efforts, however, he *did* have the power to cancel the meeting and I was not invited again until several years had passed and he had moved on to another school.

The moments that I dislike the most are when someone says, "Well, you are very good at this, but of course I can't agree with you because I am a Christian." I try to smile and say, "Oh great, I am a Christian, too." I go to church on Sundays and am an active member at the local and national levels. I don't believe that sexual health education and a belief in God are incompatible. In fact, I believe the opposite.

One of my favorite Roman Catholic priests tells people in his congregation that if they don't support sexual health education it is a sure indication that they are sexually

---

In a fourth grade classroom: "Who can tell me what the scientific name is for when the penis gets hard?"

Much muttering about hard-ons and boners. Finally, one child shoots up his hand: "I know, I know! It's called a resurrection."

immature. "Don't you dare blame your hang-ups on the church or on Christianity," he says. "Work on your own maturity." Amen.

A Worldwide Movement

The relationship between sexuality and spirituality isn't simply a concern for Christians, of course, nor is it just a modern phenomenon. In all the world's great religious traditions, there are teachings about sexuality, some thousands of years old. Many of those texts celebrate love, marriage, constancy or monogamy, and, occasionally, celibacy.

I especially admire a tale from ancient India said to be from the *Mahabharata*, of which the *Bhagavad-Gita* is a part. A young woman named Damayanti fell in love with a young man, Nala, whom she had not met but only heard about. Four chief gods tried to fool her into believing that one of them was Nala, but Damayanti chose the real Nala by noticing his sweat, dust, blinking eyes, faded garland, and by his shadow – none of which marked the perfect gods. Geoffrey Parrinder tells this story in his excellent book *Sex in the World's Religions* (General Publishing, 1980).

I am particularly fond of Damayanti because she recognized that not all love nor lovers are perfect. Yet she stayed faithful to Nala after they were married, despite many trials and transformations.

No religion says that abuse and depravity are acceptable. All teach the ideals of love, respect, and duty, as well as mutual regard and nurture. Buddha once

In a Sunday school class of six- to eight-year-olds, I was trying to explain that having sex was part of God's wonderful plan for reproduction. One child spoke up and said, "Yes, our parents have sex a lot 'cuz they love it.

A younger brother asked, "When do they do it?"

"When we stay over at Granny and Granddad's," said the older brother.

"Oh, I see," said the younger brother. "And Granny and Granddad do it when we go home again."

who made sex up?

comforted a king whose wife gave birth to a girl, saying that this child might be a greater blessing than a boy.

When I have worked with Islamic congregations they tell me about their continual study of their religious texts to understand when some of the old teachings may have been developed because of ancient conditions or misunderstandings that modern science may have made obsolete.

Of course, the same kind of study, revisiting and reinterpretation is going on among Christians and Jews. Debra W. Haffner, the remarkable past president of SIECUS (Sexual Information Education Council of the U.S.) in New York, has recently written a very comprehensive guide to sexuality education in Christian and Jewish groups. *A Time to Speak: Faith Communities and Sexuality Education* is published by SIECUS (130 West 42nd St., Suite 350, New York, NY 10036–7802). I recommend it highly to families and faith communities who want to integrate sexuality and spirituality into their lives.

I have just finished teaching students at an elementary school in Vancouver where 80 percent of the students come from a variety of immigrant cultures. Their parents had been invited to a meeting with several interpreters, but only a handful of parents attended. Those who did were very encouraging, though, and they insisted that I should visit every classroom from kindergarten through seventh grade.

All that week, as I moved through four classrooms each day, parents arrived to watch me teach. Many said, "I am so glad you are teaching my children. I cannot talk easily with them at home; my traditional religion or culture is closed on sexuality, but I learned a lot today and I want my children to learn much more than I did."

These parents recognize that the world can be much more dangerous today and that lives can be in jeopardy. One Chinese mother said it all, I think, when she said, "This lesson is not only life-saving, but it is life enhancing."

A Cambodian father told me how much he appreciated me teaching hygiene, especially washing one's genitals. He feels, rightly, I think, that we in North America have overprivatized the genitals with our anti-abuse education and the children are afraid to look at themselves. But in his religion, everyone is expected to honor the entire body and wash the genitals, not wipe blindly after using the toilet. He was thrilled when I encouraged the children to look at their genitals in the bath and to wash them regularly.

Comprehensive sexual heath education is new for all of us and we are often afraid to encourage it in our immigrant communities. We shouldn't be. I hear fifth-generation Irish Catholics, seventh-generation European Protestants, and newly arrived Africans all saying, "In my day, this was taboo."

I remember laughing with a Portuguese mom and a Greek father who both said that they had discovered that their vision of "home" had become set in cement on this topic, especially. Both confessed that when they heard about sexual health education they had thought, "This would never happen in Portugal or Greece." Yet when they returned to the "old country" last year, lo and behold, there were Greek and Portuguese schools and churches teaching sexual health and spirituality. Welcome to a worldwide movement!

Sexuality and Spirituality

Dr. David Schnarch was, until 1996, a professor of Psychiatry and Urology at the University of New Orleans. Currently, he is director of The Marriage and Family Health Center in Evergreen, Colorado. Dr. Schnarch has written a wonderful book about spirituality and sexuality called *Constructing the Sexual Crucible*. I would like to paraphrase, in point form, some of what David says in his book.

1. God is love and people's inherent capacity for love organizes human existence. Love is seen as the highest response of which we are capable, the highest moral achievement which makes community possible. Love is the moral norm by which sexual

acts are measured. Sexuality which is loving is characterized by several features:

- Investment in the partner as an individual rather than solely as a means of sexual gratification;
- Fidelity to promises and agreements;
- Mutual interest in types of sexual play;
- Non-injury to the partner;
- Responsibility for one's actions and for the well-being of the partner. It maintains concern for the significant other, the partner, the family, and society.

2. Sexual potential is part of the goodness within us. If people had more faith in themselves and in their spirituality, it would change the face of sexuality as we know it.
3. Most people do not believe what they believe they believe.
4. Loving is not for the weak. In the process of loving someone, something wondrous and awful happens. *The partner becomes unique!*

I have worked with almost every Protestant and Catholic denomination around the issues of sexual health. I have worked with many Jewish groups in Jewish schools and synagogues. I have worked with Muslim faith groups, and with people who shun any association with organized religion altogether, but who still call themselves spiritual beings. I have also worked with Christian communities who allegedly have been invaded by Satanists. That was truly the hardest work I have ever done. But knowledge is light, and education the path out of darkness. It sounds preachy, but it works.

All of us want health to be present in our own sexual relationships. Even more, we want health and sexual maturity for our young people. We may differ on semantics (the words we use), or on sacred scriptures, but the goals are the same.

All of the great religions of the world may have to acknowledge some historical shame and guilt for unhealthy sexual teaching and injunctions, as well as for sexist, homophobic, or misogynist practices. We need to recognize that many of these very hurtful things were based on ancient beliefs, political events, and plain ordinary ignorance of human biology.

Today we *can* move beyond that ignorance and bigotry. We can embrace faith precepts that are life-giving and life enhancing, and that help us celebrate the overwhelming generosity and diversity of creation. We must not continue to bring darkness and shame to the world. We must bring light! Not only that, we must *promote* light!

Does your faith community talk about sexual health at all? Ever? Do you have programs to help parents, children, teens, and seniors talk about sexuality and spirituality? Does your faith group grapple regularly with wider community issues such as reproductive technologies, sexual orientation, divorce, AIDS, or sexual health education in schools?

If you are a parent and a member of a faith group, do you talk with your children and teens about faithfulness and sexuality? Do you talk *often?* Do you follow the spiritual teachings yourself as a model for your children?

Why Bother?

When I talk to groups of young people in public schools, there is often a wonderful moment when one or two young people speak up and say, "In my religion, we believe..." Frequently, that very wise and healthful statement makes the non-religious children envious. They will say, "You are so lucky. My parents don't care (about me), they don't give me guidelines. We don't have rules at our house." The inference is, "I don't know who I am or what I am supposed to do." These children live in a vacuum or in chaos. They may not hear anything that is especially damaging or perverted, but they don't hear anything positive either. They don't hear that sexuality should be celebrated, that there is a beauty, an elegance, to it all. They don't hear that there are rights and responsibilities and choices. They don't hear that we are not simply biological creatures, at the mercy of our hormonal urges. (Many adults are stuck with this belief, too.)

There is a spiritual hunger in our world and we all need to struggle to become spiritually mature persons as well as sexually mature persons. We need to help our faith groups engage in that work as well.

IS SEX SOMETHING TO PLEASE ABOUT?

IS sex really all that good?

For Educators and Other Professionals

14

Sexual-Health Education in a Multicultural Society

I have been very fortunate and felt enormously privileged to work for many years in an area of Canada that has a long tradition of welcoming people from all over the world. Many of our ethnic communities are over 100 years old. The Chinese, Japanese, and people from the Indian subcontinent were initially involved in farming, lumbering, and building the railroads beginning in the 1800s. Some from those groups are now fourth and fifth generation Canadians. Some have managed to keep their cultural traditions and beliefs intact and some feel assimilated.

Canada has generally encouraged a cultural mosaic approach in our society and, especially in the last 40 years, ethnic groups have been encouraged to maintain their cultural identity.

Fortunately, for me, an eighth generation Anglo-Canadian, who only speaks English, this respect for our cultural mosaic means that our schools and institutions are quite accustomed to providing translators and interpreters, so let's look at some strategies for encouraging non-English speakers to attend sexual-health education sessions.

First and perhaps most obviously, notices of the meeting or workshop need to go out or to be posted in whatever languages are appropriate. Secondly, those notices need to be worded in a way that welcomes parents, that clearly states the purpose but does not intimidate anyone. Many new Canadians (and some "old" Canadians) can feel that they lack enough education themselves, to be comfortable attending such a session.

Next, an enthusiastic and supportive interpreter for each language-group is necessary. He or she should be invited to listen to a presentation first, as an audience member. This gives them the opportunity to know exactly what will be discussed, to research the scientific vocabulary or sign for the deaf and hard of hearing in their own language and to ask any questions before going before an audience to interpret. Interestingly, although interpretation has often been offered for the children's presentation, parents have always said, "No, I want my children to hear the body-science lesson in English."

I think that I can truthfully say that I have never had a parent who has attended one of my adult presentations refuse to have their child attend the family or classroom presentations.

One caution for other educators is not to be discouraged if only a few people attend the first few sessions. I have found that it sometimes takes a few years to get a sizeable part of an ethnic community to respond. Word of mouth is often the best way to encourage participation.

Don't forget that although the sexual-health education may be aimed at the children, the adults are learning life-saving information too. One heart-warming award that was given in Vancouver recently went to Dr. Lorna Sent. She discovered that Chinese women in British Columbia were getting cervical cancer at four times the rate of the general population and so she established a clinic especially for Asian women.

Considering that cervical cancer is most commonly caused by the STD called HPV, how many Asian men need this education? And how many lives could be saved by educating their children, especially boys, who are sometimes left out of the sexual-health education.

Fears of Ethnic Community

When people from conservative countries come to North America, they see sexual innuendo being used to sell everything on the billboards, in magazines and on TV, they often think that Canadians and Americans are sex mad! Naturally, they fear that we educators are going to say "sex is great, have it as much as possible." The most comforting and encouraging news that they hear from me is that we're not sex-mad, it only looks that way on TV, and that our education is about science, health, and safety. We talk about sexual activity as an adult activity and we always encourage children to talk to their families about family values and cultural norms, when we say, "Some families believe that you should be married before you have sex."

Co-ed Classes

Many ethnic parents (and some conservative religious parents) have asked me to teach the boys and girls separately. One fear is that the students will be too shy to ask questions if they are together. I always make time for anonymous written questions and everyone writes something on their paper to hand in.

Another fear is that boys and girls will learn things about each other that are inappropriate or not necessary for them to know about the opposite gender. I cannot think of one thing that fits that fear. So I reiterate that we are teaching scientific knowledge of the body, health habits that will not only serve the child but also serve well when they become adults and especially when and if they become parents.

I think that it is very poor modeling to separate boys and girls, but most of all, I know that they behave better when they are together. The boys' level of maturity rises to meet the girls'; there is much less giggling and shyness and much more participation when they are together. Standards of acceptable behavior are easier to encourage in a co-ed class.

Issues of Ethnic Communities

Children from ethnic communities are often part of large extended families and I love the groups of grandparents waiting to walk or drive children home from school, all having a great time chatting with their friends and neighbors while they wait. Of course, throughout history, grandparents have told children stories and many students have put up their hands and said, "My granddad told me…" Sometimes it is words of wisdom so wise that it brings tears to my eyes, but sometimes it is a story that is not possible or information that is very old-fashioned, or it may even be unsafe information.

Then I have to say, very carefully and gently, that grandparents didn't get body-science lessons when they were growing up and that maybe the student could share the new scientific information that we have today with the grandparent and be a body-science teacher when they get home. I do this as quickly and succinctly as I can because I don't want the rest of the class to dwell on this and open the student to teasing at recess. Then I try to move on to something else as quickly as possible.

The contentious issues for ethnic communities are likely to be the ones that are hot-button issues for all communities – homosexuality, same-sex marriage (and divorce), same-sex parenting, transgender issues, bisexuality, abortion, sex abuse, adoption, prostitution, and AIDS.

Again, as educators, we emphasize that we are teaching science, health, and safety in the classroom and encouraging the adults in all communities to become educated and aware. Cultural values and ethics can still be honored, especially those that encourage basic human rights and responsibilities, but traditions of taboo and silence are not protecting our children.

Privacy ideas about bodies and nudity in the home is an issue for some ethnic groups and again, I say, your body is not supposed to be a secret from yourself, but each family can set their own boundaries for the home.

Japan

I have been teaching sexual health in Japan for five years now and my experience with students, parents, and professionals there echoes my experience with all ethnic groups in Canada and the USA. Everyone has the same questions and the same concerns.

There are some cultural differences of course; the Japanese family sometimes sleeps together in the same room, so privacy may be a bigger issue there.

Talking about sexual health is a newer idea in Japan but I remind my Japanese audiences that we only began teaching "body-science" in Canada in the last 30 years. We are all pioneers!

Topics such as homosexuality and transgender or inter-sex issues were taboo when I began teaching, but I found that parents, students, and professionals all wanted to be more educated about the taboos and were desperate to end the silence. Sexual abuse was a terrible problem mainly, I think, because of the tradition of saving face. If the abuser was exposed, his family or his workplace would be exposed too. Fortunately, the victim's well-being is beginning to be supported and children are no longer being exploited and abused in silent communities.

AIDS has been a door-opener to sexual-health education in many countries around the world. My books have been translated and published in Russian, Romanian, Chinese, Japanese, and in India; all countries beset by AIDS and other STDs. It is very sad that it has taken a fatal or chronic disease to end taboos and silence, but with openness and education, we can end the scourge of AIDS and STDs too.

Conclusion: Celebrating Diversity

An amazing thing happens when two people decide to create a family – each child turns out differently!

Some are born with private personalities. They can be very easy to talk *to*, but they rarely give anything of themselves. Several moms have told me that they thought they had wonderful, open relationships with their daughters, that they were able to talk about everything. Then mom discovers that her daughter has been menstruating for months without telling. Mom is devastated.

"Why couldn't you tell me?"

The daughter replies with genuine puzzlement. "Why *should* I tell you? You've explained it often enough and I know all about it. *And you know, Mom, it's private!*"

Other children are born shy on the topic of sexual health. I don't know why that is, but these children never ask questions on this topic. They may ask a thousand questions about rockets or dinosaurs, but not a single one about body science.

These are children you talk *at*, constantly, grabbing every teachable moment, ignoring their silence or pained expressions. Talk the talk. Never give up or allow yourself to remain silent. When they are 30 years old, they will thank you and heap blessings on your head. You will have to wait for the thanks, but I promise you will eventually receive it.

Then there are those babies, thankfully more and more of them with each new generation, who come with hearts and minds that are wide open. They never shut up. They ask questions constantly and are fascinated by most things, including body science. They will post a list of puberty changes on the fridge and be prepared to check off things as they happen. Thank God for such children. They drag us all into greater sexual maturity and they give permission to everyone else to ask questions and to be curious.

Each child may need to be taught and guided in a different way. Some love to talk, some love books, some really appreciate videos, some need it all.

Each child is unique, a gift to our community. And as the African proverb says, "It takes a whole village to raise a child."

Let's talk the talk and get going.

Resources/Bibliography

– RESOURCES FOR PRESCHOOLERS –

Brown, Laurie Krasny, and Marc Brown. *What's the Big Secret?* New York: Little, Brown & Co., 1997. A superb book for preschoolers and primaries, all about bodies and reproduction.

Hickling, Meg. *Boys, Girls, and Body Science: A First Book about Facts of Life*. Madeira Park, BC: Harbour Publishing Co. Ltd., 2002. In this delightful picture book, Meg teams with award-winning artist Kim La Fave to re-create one of her famous body science discussions in a typical primary grade classroom. Young children learn what they need to know about sexual health in the form of a fun-to-read story.

Mayle, Peter. *Where Did I Come From?* Secaucus, NJ: Lyle Stuart Inc., 1973. This book has been around since 1973 and is still very popular, probably because of wonderful, colorful cartoon pictures. Some families love the video version which is now available.

These books tell a straightforward story of sexual health and reproduction. There are others in bookstores and libraries that tell the facts differently, but perhaps better, for some families. Choose the ones that feel most comfortable for you. Read them first to yourself, then share them with your spouse or with others who care for your child.

Remember that you don't have to read every word of the text to your child the first time – just talk about the pictures until you get more comfortable.

No book will ever be perfect, but every book will start a discussion. Don't be afraid to say "I don't agree with this part," or "I'd put this part differently," or "I wish that the book talked about..."

Books and videos can be great tools for children and their families. Children often need to go back again and again to get the facts straight, to accept them, and finally to integrate them. Be prepared to repeat, reread, and re-teach.

Sexual Abuse –
to be read after the health information books above

There is a host of books, tapes, videos, coloring books, and puppet kits to teach preschoolers about privacy and to say "no-go-tell" when they are approached in an inappropriate manner.

I would advise parents to look at as many as possible and to choose the one or two that you feel most comfortable with and able to use. Try to choose the resource that gives you the greatest spread of options for talking. Please don't stay with "stranger-danger" material. Most abusers of preschoolers are family members or caregivers.

You will want to teach your child that it is okay to say "no" to an older person and to tell on that person.

Remember that peer abuse or exploitation is also possible, so that if the parent dwells on strangers as abusers, the child is far from empowered.

Hindman, Jan. *The Very Touching Book*. Ontario, OR: Alexandria, 1990. This is my very favorite book for preschoolers and their families. It has lots of hilarious pictures, it is non-threatening, and children of all ages just love it.

Adoption

There are now many more books available than ever before, some especially for very young children. Again, look at them all, or as many as you can find in stores and in libraries. Don't forget to check with your local or national adoption agencies for recommendations. There are also books for multiracial adoptions.

Carlson, Nancy. *My Family Is Forever*. New York: Viking Books, 2004.
A heart-warming story with lovely illustrations.

Lewis, Rose A. *I Love You Like Crazy Cakes*. New York: Little Brown, 2000.

HIV/AIDS

As some babies are born HIV positive, and as more of them live longer, we must be prepared to meet them in preschools.

Merrifield, Dr. Margaret. *Come Sit by Me*. Toronto: Women's Press, 1990. This is one of the very nicest books for families and preschoolers. It is like a preschooler's storybook with lots of gorgeous color pictures. It tells the story of a preschool that has an HIV-positive child attending. I cannot recommend this book too highly. It deals with the subject in a non-frightening way. There is plenty of small-print information for parents too. Also on video.

Merrifield, Dr. Margaret. *Morning Light*. Toronto: Stoddart, 1995. This book is for young children and talks about parents who are HIV positive. Again, it is beautifully done and deals with a tragedy in a most helpful way.

– RESOURCES FOR PRIMARIES –

If your child has not had a book on sexual health issues before, you may want to begin with a book from the preschool list. None of those listed is too "babyish" for a primary student. Then, once the very basic facts and vocabulary are established, you will want resources that are more sophisticated.

You might want to provide a book of body science that explores the whole body plus the reproductive system and topics related to sexual health. There are many excellent books available with pop-ups, fold-outs, transparencies, and dazzling graphics. Primaries love to know the mechanical details of digestion (especially "poo" and "pee"), respiration, blood circulation, and so on.

There are a number of superb, almost comic-style books on body science published by Usborne in Britain and available worldwide.

Abramchik, Lois. *Is Your Family Like Mine?* Brooklyn: Open Mind, Open Heart, 1993. A marvelous, small book that helps primaries recognize and appreciate all kinds of family constellations, including foster families.

Stones, Rosemary. *Where Do Babies Come From?* New York: Puffin Books, 1989. This book has great, colorful illustrations showing diversity of ethnic groups. The text is very matter-of-fact and easy to read. A relatively inexpensive paperback book.

Harris, Robie. *It's So Amazing: A Book about Eggs, Sperm, Birth, Babies, and Families*. Cambridge, MA: Candlewick Press, 1999. A multi-award winning book for young children and their caregivers. Dr. A. F. Poussaint from Harvard's faculty of psychiatry called it "a book every family should own."

The following are some Japanese books in translation which satisfy primaries' fascination with elimination. I recommend them, but only for those with a sense of humor.

Cho, Shinto. *The Gas We Pass*. Brooklyn: Kane/Miller Book Publishers, 1978.

Gomi, Taro. *Everyone Eats and Poops*. Brooklyn: Kane/Miller Book Publishers, 1977.

Nanao, Jun. *Contemplating Your Belly Button*. Brooklyn: Kane/Miller Book Publishers, 1995.

Beginning Puberty

It is always a good idea to introduce the topic of puberty changes to primary students before the changes begin. This prepares the family to keep talking all the way through puberty and it tells the child that it is appropriate to confide in the parent. And remember, it's always easier to laugh and relax *before* puberty starts.

Bourgeois, P., and M. Wolfish. *Changes in You and Me*. Toronto: Somerville, 1994. There are two versions of this book, one "Mostly for Girls" and one "Mostly for Boys." They are almost identical and have transparent pages which intrigue children. They give factual information and are simply written.

Harris, Robie. *It's Perfectly Normal*. Cambridge, MA: Candlewick Press, 1994. This is a very comprehensive look at puberty with marvelous illustrations. It has a pair of comedians – a bird and a bee – who wisecrack their way through the book and add a great deal of welcome humor. This is an especially good book for keen readers, aged 8 and up.

Mayle, Peter. *What's Happening To Me?* New York: Carol Publishing Group, 1975. The funniest book ever about puberty with cartoon pictures and a humorous text that introduces puberty changes in a very simple way. Available on video.

Understanding Homosexuality and Diversity

Books to help children understand orientation and to help parents explain diverse families, alternative living styles, and all the "out of the closet" ways of being human that children see on the afternoon talk shows, are only just beginning to be published. There are a few good ones.

de Haan, Linda, and Stern Nijland. *King & King*. Berkeley: Tricycle Press, 2002. Also *King & King & Family*. Berkeley: Tricycle Press, 2004. These two books are very funny fairy tales with great illustrations. They tell the story of homosexual orientation without naming it as such, just celebrating diversity. Suitable for ages three to 103.

Elwin, Rosamund, and Michele Paulse. *Asha's Mums*. Toronto: Women's Press, 1990. This book is written for primary children and is very well done. It tells the story of a girl and her brother in a family with two mums. There are multiracial children in the illustrations and many younger children will recognize classroom discussions.

Galloway, Priscilla. *Jennifer Has Two Daddies*. Toronto: Women's Press, 1985. A more sophisticated story than *Asha's Mums*, but again, very well done. It has marvelous illustrations.

Manasse, Geoff, and Jean Swallow. *Making Love Visible: In Celebration of Gay and Lesbian Families*. Freedom, CA: The Crossing Press, 1995. A welcome book filled with marvelous photos and interviews with a diverse group of families. One reviewer calls it "hymns to the spirit of family." This softcover book would be especially useful for parents and children who live in gay and lesbian families in smaller towns where pride and acceptance are not always visible.

Simon, Norma. *All Families Are Special.* Morton Grove, IL: Albert Whitman & Company, 2003. Young children tell their teacher about their families, which are all different.

Tax, Meredith. *Families*. New York: The Feminist Press, 1996. Multi-ethnic or multiconfiguration families are celebrated.

– RESOURCES FOR INTERMEDIATES –

Any of the books listed in the previous two sections could be a great starting place for children aged eight to 14 who have not yet had any sexual health education.

Once the basics are established, there are more sophisticated and challenging books to move to, usually to be read by the child in private. These shy intermediates will often accept a book and read it avidly if it is given to them by a favorite adult or older teen. That makes it much more acceptable than if the same book comes from a parent!

Gurian, Michael. *From Boys to Men*. New York: Price, Stern, Sloan, 1999. A small book for boys with a super chapter called "What's Happening to Your Mind?" to help with puberty and adolescence.

McCoy, Kathy, and Charles Wibbelsman, M.D. *Growing and Changing: A Handbook for Preteens.* New York: Perigee, 1986. This is a large format paperback book with honest answers to hundreds of typical preteen questions. It deals with physical and emotional changes and is great for parents to read as well. Reissued in 2003 in a newer format – a classic.

Schaefer, Valorie, et. al. *The Care and Keeping of You: The Body Book for Girls*. Middleton, WI: American Girl Library, Pleasant Company Publications, 1998.The most wonderful book for girls aged 7-14 about puberty, with the best illustrations.

Siegel, Peggy C. *Changes in You for Boys* and *Changes in You for Girls*. Richmond, VA: Family Life Education Associates (PO. Box 7466, Richmond, Virginia, 23221), 1992. There are two books, one for girls and one for boys, written especially for children who may be intellectually challenged or developmentally delayed. Both books contain Parents' Guides. Available in the U.S.

A Word to the Wise

One very nervous father told me that he and his 12-year-old son had been browsing in a bookstore when his son asked him if he would buy him *The Male Sexual Machine: An Owner's Manual* by Kenneth Purvis, M.D., Ph.D. (New York: St. Martin's Press, 1992).

The father hesitated but, bless him, he did buy it for his son. He wanted to know if I thought that he had acted appropriately. I could have hugged him. First, what a wonderful compliment that the boy felt so comfortable asking for the book, and second, that the dad bought it for him. This is also a great book for a teenager who will read it just because of its wacky title.

This is a superb book for males of all ages and is written in a straightforward, easy-to-read style. I love the way the stories are set out in boxes.

Single parents often feel that they cannot talk to their opposite-sex child. Books might be a great way for both parent and child to embark on a learning journey. Don't forget that even same-sex parents don't know it all and that books can keep you modern!

A good book for females in their later intermediate years, and their parents, would be *The New Our Bodies, Ourselves* by the Boston Women's Health Book Collective (New York: Touchstone, 1992) and I like *A New View of a Woman's Body* by the Federation of Feminist Women's Health Centers (West Hollywood, CA: Feminist Health Press, 1991).

No intermediate, and probably no adult, would sit down and read these books from cover to cover. They are meant to be read as a resource, in small sections, as the need for information arises.

Sexual Abuse

Intermediates experience the highest incidence of sexual abuse, perhaps because abusers tend to abuse victims who are the same age as they were when they were abused.

There are some very useful books for families who are trying to help their abused children. Here are a few.

Hagans, Kathryn B., and Joyce Case. *When Your Child Has Been Molested: A Parent's Guide to Healing and Recovery*. New York: Jossey-Bass, 1988.

Jessie. *Please Tell: A Child's Story About Sexual Abuse*. Hazelden, 1991. Written and illustrated by Jessie.

Satullo, Jane, Roberta Russell, and Pat A. Bradway. *It Happens to Boys Too*. Published by the Rape Crisis Center of Berkshire County, 18 Charles St., Pittsfield, MA, 01201, USA, 1992.

Sometimes, when a child is victimized by abuse and doesn't receive effective treatment, they become sexually intrusive themselves. And bullying is another problem intermediates face. Here are two helpful books, one on each topic.

Cavanagh Johnson, Toni. *Understanding Your Child's Sexual Behavior*. Oakland, CA: New Harbinger Publications, 1991.

— *Helping Children with Sexual Behavior Problems: A Guidebook for Parents and Substitute Caregivers*. Self-published. 1101 Fremont Ave., Suite 101, South Pasadena, CA 91030, USA.

Kaufman, Gershen, and Lev Raphael. *Stick Up for Yourself*. Minneapolis: Free Spirit, 1990. Revised in 1999. This book can be read and shared by families who want to arm their intermediates before they are bullied, but also during or after a bullying situation. It can be used as a workbook too and is extremely well laid out.

– RESOURCES FOR ADOLESCENTS –

Bell, Ruth (with members of the Teen Book Project). *Changing Bodies, Changing Lives*. New York: Vintage Books, 1992. This is a perennial favorite, a large paperback which answers many questions.

Girlsource editorial team. *Girl Source: A Book by and for Young Women about Relationships, Rights, Futures*. Berkeley: Tricycle Press, 2003.

Jukes, Mavis. *The Guy Book: An Owner's Manual for Teens*. New York: Crown Books for Young Readers, 2002. This book is done like a car manual: "Safety, maintenance, and operating instructions."

Any book written for adults about healthy sexuality and sexually mature relationships can be read by teens. They need time to absorb the information, decide where their own boundaries will be, and make informed decisions. It is sad that so many teens are "informed" by pornography instead!

One of the newest and most impressive books that provides an encyclopedic overview of sexuality in all its areas is *Reader's Digest Guide to Love and Sex*, consulting editors, Dr. Amanda Roberts, and Dr. Barbara Padget-Yawn, 1998.

– RESOURCES FOR PARENTS –

Many people start to learn about sexuality, sexual health, and health in general when they become adults and parents themselves. Some excellent books to start you off, or to bring you up to date, have been published lately. Remember that there are always new things being discovered and therefore new things to learn. Learning is really a lifelong task.

Arnold, Jeanne. *Amy Asks a Question: Grandma, What's a Lesbian?* Racine, WI: Mother Courage Press, 1996. This book, about Amy and the coolest grandma, is designed to help adults explain homosexuality and homophobia to children. I recommend it to all adults and especially to cool grandmas.

Coloroso, Barbara. *Kids Are Worth It: Giving Your Child the Gift of Inner Discipline*. New York: HarperResource, 2002.

DeMarco, Carolyn. *Take Charge Of Your Body; Women's Health Advisor*. Toronto: Well Woman Press, 1994. Super for girls and women.

Hister, Art. *Midlife Man: A Not-So-Threatening Guide to Health & Sex for Man at His Peak*. Vancouver: Greystone Books, 1998.

Meyer, Chuck. *Twelve Smooth Stones: A father writes to his daughter about sex, money, spirituality, and other things that really matter.* Kelowna, BC: Northstone Publishing, 1999. These wise and witty letters cover everything from alcohol and drugs, to sex, money, work, spiritual beliefs, pornography, and dying; and model great parent-teen communication.

Morgentaler, A. *The Male Body: What Every Man Should Know about His Sexual Health.* New York: Simon and Schuster, 1993.

Taguchi, Y. *Private Parts: An Owner's Guide.* Toronto: McClelland & Stewart, 1988.

– RESOURCES FOR CHRISTIAN FAMILIES –

The following three books are all published under the auspices of The Lutheran Church, Missouri Synod for Christian Families. They are very well done and offer a refreshing approach. Consider this sentence: "What a miracle of God the scrotum and testicles are." All I can say is, "Right On!"

Bimler, Richard. *Sex and the New You: Ages 11–14.* St. Louis, Missouri: Concordia Publishing House, 1995.

Buth, Lenore. *How to Talk Confidently with Your Child about Sex and Appreciate Your Own Sexuality Too: Parents Guide.* St. Louis: Concordia Publishing House, 1995.

Graver, Jane. *How You Are Changing: Ages 8-11 and Parents.* St. Louis: Concordia Publishing House, 1995.

Here are some other titles.

Gordon, Sol, and Judith Gordon. *Raising a Child Conservatively in a Sexually Permissive World.* New York: Simon and Schuster, 1983. An excellent book written from a Judeo-Christian viewpoint, with down-to-earth guidance for parents.

Miller, Patricia M. *Sex Is Not a Four-Letter Word.* New York: Crossroad, 1994. A superb book with up-to-date information for parents who want to talk with their children and communicate thoughtful Christian values.

– RESOURCES FOR PARENTS OF CHILDREN WITH DISABILITIES –

The following agencies can provide or suggest great resources for parents of children with disabilities.

Sexual Health Resource Network
 Library, B. C. Children's Hospital
 4480 Oak St.
 Vancouver, BC V6H 3V4
 Phone: 604-875-2345
 www.cw.bc.ca

National Information Center for Children and Youth with Disabilities
 (NICHCY)
 P.O. Box 1492
 Washington, DC 20013-1492
 Phone/TTY: 1-800-695-0285 Fax: 202-884-8441
 Website: http://www.nichcy.org

– WEBSITES –

www.sieccan.org

> Sex Information & Education Council of Canada. A starting place to learn more about sexuality. Includes information on the Canadian Guidelines and common questions about sexuality education.

www.familiesaretalking.org

> Sex Information & Education Council of the United States. The American SIECCUS site with more information about talking with children about sexuality.

Index

A

abortion 174
abuse
  homophobia 67
  homosexuality 150
  protection against 29, 63, 77, 155
  sexual-health education 33, 37
  sleep disturbances 99
  STDs 173
  untreated 76
abusive relationships 100, 124
adult sexual maturity
  definition of 124
AIDS (acquired immune deficiency
    syndrome) 178
  for primaries 68
  homosexuality 152
  lifestyles 147
  pornography 160
alcohol
  birth control, pill and, 115, 174
amniotic fluid 47
anal sex 157, 158
analgesics
  birth control, pill and, 115, 174
andropause 127
antacids
  birth control, pill and, 115, 174
antibiotics
  birth control, pill, 115, 174
antihistamines
  birth control, pill, 115, 174
anus 43, 47
  hemorrhoids 101
  medical examinations 192
  STDs 152, 159

are you ready for sex
  checklist 172
arousal in children 45

B

bathing
  nudity in the home 156
bedtime sharing 27, 71
birth control
  condoms 114
  family values 203
  for teens 114
  IUDs (intrauterine devices) 114
  morning-after pill 116
  myths
    bathing, hot tubs, etc. 116
    cola 116
    first time is free 117
    menstruation 117
    standing up 116
  outercourse 118
  sponges 114
  the pill 114
    decreased effectiveness 115, 173
  STDs 114
bisexual 151
blow job 157
body image 93
breast
  budding 70
  cancer
    in males 124
    pubertal changes and fear 82
  development in pubertal boys 82
  medical examinations 196
  milk production 84

self-examination 124
size 84, 165
soreness 83
bust enlargers 165

C

calcium 90
cancer
   breast
      pubertal changes and fear 82
   male breast 124
   medical examinations 195
   STDs, liver 181
   testicular 88, 124, 151
cervix 195
Cesarean or C-section 48, 61, 186
child pornography 160
chlamydia 147, 182
circumcision 40, 41
clitoris 45
conception 30, 81, 100, 176
      alternative 134, 136
condoms 53
   birth control 114
   penis size 170
   STDs for intermediates 100
contraception. *See* birth control
contraceptives
   decreased effectiveness 115, 173
contractions 48
cross-dressing 163, 164

D

dating 201
depression 94
digital sex/fingering 157
dildo 165
disabilities
   and sex 147
disabled children 30, 239

discipline 110
divorce 99

E

ectopic pregnancies 184
emotional development
      adolescents 93
endometrium 89
erections 39
      male menopause 127
      urination 39

F

family values
   birth control 203
   dating 201
   pornography 202
   television 213
fingering/digital sex 157
foreskin
   circumcision 42
   genital warts 182
   hygiene 40
   smegma 44

G

genital herpes 186
genital warts 181
      medical examinations 192
gonorrhea 182
grandparents
   as teachers 26

H

hemorrhoids 101
hepatitis 54
   B and C 181
   vaccination 118
heterosexism 146

heterosexual
  homophobia 151
  propositioning by homosexuals 153
heterosexuality
  cross-dressing 164
  medical examinations 191, 194
  STDs 152, 179
  types of sex 151
HIV (human immunodeficiency virus)
    178
  AIDS for Primaries 69
homophobia 146, 151, 153
  suicide 150, 151
homosexuality 149
  cross-dressing 164
  marriages 146
hormones
  emotional development 93
  homosexuality 150
  testosterone 42
    male menopause 127
human papilloma virus (HPV) 181
hygiene
  at puberty 84
  vulva 89
hymen 194
hysterectomy 125, 129

I

impotence 119
in vitro fertilization. *See* test-tube
    babies
Internet
  pornography 208

J

jaundice, hepatitis 181

L

labia 44

M

magnesium 90
male climacteric 127
male menopause 127
masturbation 155
mechanical curiosity 72
menopause 129
  perimenopause 129
menstruation
  cramps 90
  for intermediates 89
  for preschoolers 50
  for primaries 70
  menopause 129
  vegetarianism 90
  who should explain 25
miscarriage 80
mucous membrane 159
multicultural issues 223

N

nausea, hepatitis 181
navel 48, 49
nipple
  breast budding 70
  soreness 83
nocturnal emissions
  for intermediates 92
  for preschoolers 52
  for primaries 70
  who should explain 25
nudity
  bathing 156
  embarrassment 78
  in the home 77, 156
  sleeping in the nude 42

O

oral sex 157
orgasm 148
  in infants 45, 155
  teen sex 106
ova
  fraternal twins 81
ovaries 41
  damage from smoking 108
  medical examination 193, 195
  torsions 42
ovum
  identical twins 81
  meets sperm 24
    preschoolers 38
    primaries 60
  menstruation 90
  STDs, ectopic pregnancies 183
  test-tube babies 135

P

pap smear 195
pelvic exam 195
penis
  damage from smoking 107
  erections 39, 155
  function 24, 39
  inappropriate touching 63
  naming 23
  sexual intercourse 22
  size 88
    enlargers 165
    function 88
    growth 87
    micropenis 88
    pornography 87
  STDs 183
    genital warts 182
  stretcher 165
PID (pelvic inflammatory disease)
  183

pornography 159
  child 160
  family values 208
  Internet 208
  suicide 160
pregnancy 81, 184
  are you ready for sex 172, 173
  homophobia 151
  making babies 47
  outercourse 118
  prevention myths 116
  sexual-health education 33
  test-tube babies 136
prostate
  infertility 183
  medical examinations 192
  STDs 183
prostitution 162
puberty 82
  hygiene 84
  pre-puberty information 69
pubic hair 85
purple nurples 92

R

rape 46
  morning-after pill 116
  sexual maturity 125
rules 110

S

"sensuous" children 62
scrotal sac 41
scrotum 41
sexuality
  and spirituality 216
sexually transmitted diseases (STDs)
  birth control and 114
  ectopic pregnancies 184
  for adults 125
  for intermediates 100

for teens 118, 170, 173
  homosexuality 152
  infertility 183
  lifestyles 147
sexual assault
  wedgies and purple nurples 92
sexual-health education
  benefits 32
sex change 163
  ovaries 164
  testicles 164
sex toys 165
  dildo 165
  vibrator 165
shy children 64
sleep 97
  disturbances 97, 99
    male menopause 127
  inducers 99
  patterns 99
smegma 44
  hygiene 85
smoking 107
speculum 194
sperm
  donor sperm 138
  fraternal and identical twins 81
  manufacture of 42
  meets ovum 24
    preschoolers 38
    primaries 60
  STDs 158
sperm banks 135
spirituality
  and sexuality 216
steroids 180
stool 43, 47
  samples 43, 192
sweat 84
syphilis 187

T

tampons 50, 51
  toxic shock syndrome 51, 152
television 162, 202
test-tube babies 135
testicles 41
  examinations 88, 191
  puberty 87
  self-examination 124
  sensitivity 37
  sperm production 52, 162
  STDs 183
  torsions 42
testicular cancer 88, 124, 151
testosterone 42
  male menopause 127, 128
toxic shock syndrome 51, 152
transgendered 163
transsexual 163
transvestite 163
tubal ligation 129
twins 97
  fraternal 99
  identical 99

U

umbilical cord 48
urethra 43
  boys 43
  girls 45
  passage of sperm 39
urination
  females 43, 183
  magical thinking 37
  males 43
  STDs 183, 186
uterus
  making babies 47
  medical examinations 193
  menstruation 50
  STDs 183
  test-tube babies 135

V

vagina 44, 45
  medical examinations 194
  naming 44
  orgasm 148
  rape or sexual assault 46
  sexual intercourse 22
  STDs 183
  test-tube babies 135
vaginal birth 59
vasectomy 125
vegetarianism
  and menstruation 90
venereal/genital warts 152
Viagra 119
vibrator 165
virgin 144
viropause 127
vitamin B12 90
voice changes 85
vulva 44
  hygiene 89
  labia 44
  naming 24
  smegma 44

W

wedgies 92
wet dreams 52, 92
where babies come from 47